THE PSYCHIATRIC TOWER OF BABBLE

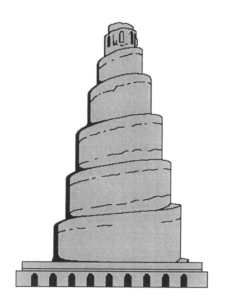

SUE GABRIEL

Diverse City Press Inc. (La Presse Divers Cité Inc.)
BM 272, 33 rue des Floralies
Eastman, Quebec
CANADA J0E 1P0

LITHO CANADA   〜〜〜 METROLITHO   Sherbrooke (Québec)

Gabriel, Susan R.
The Psychiatric Tower of Babble: Understanding People
with Developmental Disabilities who have Mental Illness.

Hanna, Mary   (illus.)

ISBN 1-896230-01-6

1. Mentally Handicapped 2. Mental Health

DEDICATION

This book is dedicated to all the people who let me share their story, and a small part of their lives.

Thanks must also be given to Fritz and Angela who gave me the time and opportunity to learn what I thought I already knew. Given my less than adequate typing and computer skills, thanks also to Cathy, Mary Lou, and especially Mary.

One beautiful summer day in the northern wilds of Canada, Dave casually asked, "Have you ever wanted to write a book?" I can't begin to thank all at Diverse City Press for turning my dream into this reality. Dave nurtured the reality, Joe laughed at my jokes while correcting my grammar, and Erin pulled this work together. Thank you.

Finally, thanks to my parents, Wally and Shirley Smith, and my husband Charlie. You weren't always sure of where I was going, but you always believed that I would get there. Maybe someday I will.

DISCLAIMER

This book is intended to help the reader gain knowledge about psychiatric disorders. It is *not* intended to provide the reader with enough information to make their own diagnosis and prescribe treatment. Assessment, diagnosis and treatment should all be completed by the appropriate licensed practitioner. Even though new information comes out about currently available medication, or medication of the future, a new edition of this book cannot come out each month to keep you, the reader, up to date. That is also the job of your mental health practitioner. On the other hand, having a handle on what information is necessary for a proper assessment, and having a basic knowledge of the expectations of treatment *can* help you or the person or persons you are concerned about.

Contents

S.S.R.I.'s, B.T.P.'s, neurotransmitters, contingency plans, psychiatrist, psychologist, prescriptions, negative consequences...HELP!

Many years ago, during my job interview with a community agency for developmental disabilities, I had to ask what "D.D." meant -- twice! Deinstitutionalization sounded like the last word in the National Spelling Bee. I couldn't help but remember my Sunday school teacher and long-time family friend try to explain God's actions in Babylon.

The Tower of Babel, Genesis 11:1, 5-9

> At first, the people of the whole world had only one language and used the same words.... Then the Lord came down to see the city and the tower which those men had built, and He said, "Now then, these are all one people and they speak one language; this is just the beginning of what they are going to do. Soon they will be able to do anything they want! Let us go down and mix up their language so that they will not understand each other." So the Lord scattered them all over the earth, and they stopped building the city. The city was called Babylon, because there the Lord mixed up the language of all the people, and from there He scattered them all over the earth.

Although my faith dictates that I accept God's actions, I don't understand it even today.

I understand even less the human service systems designed to help people with disabilities and the systems' tendencies to emulate this confusion of language. It sometimes seems that to the person entering the world of dual diagnosis (developmental disabilities with psychiatric impairment), there is no common language. Persons from the disabilities side of the fence often speak of behaviors, averages, and learned responses. Mental health staff often refer to biochemical alterations. Parents want simply to understand and help their 32 year old son who has Down Syndrome. He spends all his time in his room. He violently refuses to participate in activities that he used to love. He doesn't sleep well, he won't bathe. Welcome to the Psychiatric Tower of Babble.

This book is not designed to detail all of the research. It is not designed to cure systems attempting to assist persons with dual diagnosis. Hopefully, however, the reader will have a better understanding of the complexities involved in a language we can all understand.

In the Beginning

In the fall of 1983, the social worker sat at her desk looking at me rather incredulously. "You *want* to work with people who are retarded *and* behavior problems? Well, do I have the lady for you. Jessie is thirty-five years old. She's been on more behavior treatment plans than I can count. She swears, throws furniture and is a problem to everyone in the home. Frankly, I don't think she even has the mouth muscles to smile."

I drove and drove out to the 'community inclusive' group home located miles from anywhere to meet Jessie for the first time. Staff informed me she was in her room. "Hi Jessie, I'm Sue". She glanced at me from her bed and looked down. "Do you know why I'm here?" Now she finally acknowledged me. "Yeah. Because I'm bad." I wanted to cry. She did.

According to the National Association for the Dually Diagnosed (NADD), dual diagnosis is the combined existence of a developmental disability such as mental retardation or autism along with psychiatric impairment. Confusion often exists about these two conditions. Some believe that there is no difference between a developmental disability and a psychiatric illness. In fact, for centuries persons deemed 'different' were clustered away together. Without a diganosis, they were described using the labels of fear: they were amoral, degenerate, and in general, drains on society.

Prior to the early 1960's (and really up until about 1970) when a child with an obvious developmental disability was born, the advice given by the authorities to parents was to place the child in an institution. As a matter of fact, parents were encouraged to forget that their child had ever been born. I remember one gentlemen I met when I worked in an adult foster care home. His name was Joe. I was surprised that his younger brother's name was also Joe. It seemed that the family wanted a 'real person' to carry the name of Joe. They followed the professionals' advice and tried to forget Joe #1. I'm not sure they ever did.

It was probably even worse for those individuals with a mild impairment which wasn't quite as obvious at birth. Imagine a child who is about five or six years of age. He was a little bit slow during the pre-school years, but hey, all kids are different. Who pays a whole lot of attention to little things? When he be reached school age, he failed kindergarten or first grade. The teacher said in kind professional tones, "This kid is an idiot." Once labeled (using the language of the time) as an 'imbecile,' 'idiot,' or 'low-grade moron,' schools would refuse to teach.

"Keep him at home, or put him away, he's your problem not ours," was the message from the educational system. The parents, then, had only two choices. They could keep him at home. And, no, there would be no additional support. Or, there was another choice. The one, again, recommended by professionals was institutionalization. There were big buildings located far away from where anybody else lived. "They have doctors! They have nurses! There are even teachers! They will help your poor boy. Put him there."

It all seemed so simple, really. But here is the

clincher, 'child retardates' had a hard time 'adapting to new living situations.' Parents were informed that, "We (the professionals) will take your child. But. (And it was a big but!) But when you drop him off you are to have no contact either by phone or in person for three months, no-- six would be better, actually nine months or even a year would really help him adjust." I can't imagine what this would have done to me. When I look at my daughter, I wonder what it would do to her to be dropped off at a big building and say goodbye for a year. What would it do to her!? I wonder what the drive home would be like for me. No wonder some parents never made the drive back.

Sometimes parents were not even given the choice. Mrs. Miller greeted me with her worn out smile. I had been treating her 60 year old son who has depression. On this particular day, Mrs. Miller got a haunted, far away look in her eyes, and slowly began to speak of the day she lost her son. "I was hanging up clothes in the backyard. All three kids, were outside playing. We all knew Donald was slow and would never go to school, but I didn't care. I loved him, he was mine." She paused as if to gain more strength. With a gulp, she continued, "The sheriff's car pulled up. They had a warrant to take Donald away. The doctor in town thought Donald took too much of my time away from the other children. The doctor talked to the judge, but he never talked to me. I wasn't even allowed to get Donald a clean set of clothes. He was nine years old." She paused again, composing herself, "The next time I saw him he was twelve and looked at me as if he hated me. I hated me." At that moment, I represented the system who stole her son. I hated me too. I can still see the tears on her face.

As a psychiatric nurse practitioner, I see people diagnosed as dually diagnosed. Sometimes I meet their families. Families have been steam rolled by the system many times over. Some families I meet are angry, some are sad, some are depressed, some argue, some are 'non-compliant.' All, like Mrs. Miller, are exhausted. I understand them better now.

My husband and I have now had our own journey which began when we watched our very bright child enter first grade. She was excited about going to school and her excitement was contagious. As the months went by we slowly watched the lights of joy fade from her eyes. She knew something was 'wrong' before we were ready to examine it. When we were, we found that she had dyslexia -- a learning disability. Once tested, once labelled, I still didn't want to accept it.

My first phone call with the school after having her tested was like a slap in the face. I spoke with the principal to discuss how this information was going to effect my child's schooling. I was asked if our daughter was failing. I explained that she wasn't; in fact she was doing average work. "Well, if she's not failing, why did you even have her tested?" The prinicpal's tone was not friendly, in fact her voice could have cut a diamond. I couldn't believe it. I explained that as is typical with someone who has dyslexia, my daughter's intelligence is quite high, and the fact that she was not able to work up to her potential was our clue. Now what we wanted was reassurance from the school and help for our child. Naive, huh?

Over the past few months I've experienced (and still do!) denial. We waited months for the testing. In part because of hectic family life, but maybe because of not wanting to hear the truth. I've felt anger -- it's been all the school's fault, the teacher's fault and of course, my husband's fault -- he, after all, also has dyslexia. I've even been angry at my daughter for 'not trying hard enough.' Sometimes, I'm even mildly accepting. In those times I realize that she's still our super kid who has harder challenges in reading and writing. **BUT I DON'T LIKE IT!** I don't like how it makes me feel, I don't like how hard she has to work, and I really don't like being on the other side of the parent/professional paradigm.

For the families, I've worked with, I'm sorry for my professional arrogance in the past. One good thing about writing a book like this is I get to seek public absolution. For professionals reading this book, we need to understand families from their perspective *before* we condemn them with our professional righteousness. For parents, again, I'm sorry.

The 1960's came along and, in America, it was the time of Camelot and John F. Kennedy. A new word was about to be heard -- deinstitutionalization. John F. Kennedy's sister had mental retardation and his mother, Rose, was determined not to put her daughter in an institution. It was very fortunate that they were Kennedy's. They could create options where others had none. They could hire whomever they needed. Although (and maybe because), the President's sister was ultimately placed in an institution, the family recognized the lack of options faced by families. The Kennedy family has a history of activating social change. President Kennedy signed into law the deinstitutionalization of persons with retardation and persons with mental illness. Community Mental Health began.

By the 1970's we were starting to bring people out of institutions and create new environments. The idea that people with disabilities could live in real homes and real

5

communities is largely a tribute to the early behavior therapists. The pioneers of education for people with disabilities were those who believed that ALL could be taught. Behaviorists brought new technology and new expectations. They managed to prove *scientifically* that people with developmental disabilities could learn if someone bothered to teach them. The literature of the time was full of stories of people with disabilities who learned astounding skills in record time just for a bit of social interaction. This radically changed the picture of a 'hopelessly retarded soul' into a being that could think and learn. As people moved out, it was a come as you are ... or more aptly come as you are -- on drugs! These people were on medications but we weren't really sure if they worked, how they worked or why they worked. But, with medication and behavioral training we were able to begin the journey home.

Many people held (and still do today) that a person with a developmental disability is an eternal child within an adult body. As long as the person was cute, loveable, and compliant, movement into the community wasn't too bad. Persons with mental illness, on the other hand, were still seen as evil, amoral, and dangerous.

I can remember learning in my psychiatric nursing course at the University of Michigan in the late 1970's that the probable cause of schizophrenia was poor parenting -- strong mom, weak dad, and 'double-bind' communications. The medications were called 'Major Tranquilizers' as compared to Valium which was a 'Minor Tranquilizer'. The idea was that the person with schizophrenia was so 'anxious' that the anxiety caused the ambivalence, the turning away from people, and even the paranoia. The delusions and hallucinations were 'non functional' coping strategies. It never made sense to me that there could be that many messed up families.

During my student nurse rotation at the state psychiatric hospital, I was frightened most of the time I was there. Unfortunately, fear didn't count when you had paper assignments to complete. One of our assignments (infinitely more useful for me than the patient) was a 'process recording.' We were to record a five minute conversation (on paper) with a patient. My subject was Carol. Carol was forty-seven. She had been living at the state hospital for more years than I'd been on this earth. Our five-minute conversation focused on Carol's need to brush her teeth. It had been so long since she had brushed her teeth, no one (myself included) really wanted to talk to her. Carol's needs, confusion, and fears didn't relate to anything I'd learned in class. I had to wing it on my own -- with her help. I just knew that if Carol tried hard enough, I'd be able to find out the rest of her problems, cure her and leave her with sparkling white teeth. I got a 'B' in the class. I didn't cure her. I did finally bring her a new toothbrush from home, but it was never used by the time the semester ended. I never wanted to return.

As my experiences at the psych hospital paralleled general social beliefs, I had no trouble believing that retarded people were sweet and kind. They were certainly not like 'those people'. 'Those people' were hopeless. 'My people' were always going to need guidance by special people like myself.

My husband and I recently bought a cottage not far from the group home where I worked when I met Joe. Although Joe has since passed away, many people from the home that I knew fifteen years ago are still living in that town. This past Easter, I was thrilled to see several of them in church. I thought to re-introduce myself so they could feel 'accepted by the normal people' (As you can see, I still have a lot to learn). Frankly, I couldn't get near them because of their friends. A former staff person meant little to them -- much, much less than seeing them meant to me. I left humbled and excited.

After I graduated with my shiny new diploma from the University of Michigan, I worked in regular community hospitals. It was there I had a major self-realization -- I hated working midnights and weekends. After eight months of looking like a survivor from "Night of the Living Dead", I joined the waking world. I became a nurse for a community agency in Detroit, Michigan, serving people with developmental disabilities. This was the early 1980's and the term 'D.D.' was brand new. We had a full staff of 'behaviorals.' They were vital because not all clients (no longer called patients!) were sweet and kind. More and more people being released from institutions had a wide variety of 'negative behavior' learned in 'negative settings.' The behaviorists had worked miracles in the institution, why not here?

The fundamental belief of behaviorism at the time it was taught to me, is that 'man' is an empty box. There are no internal drives, emotions, and personalities that are not a direct result from outside influences. They explained that the same two parents could produce three completely different people because of different exposures and expectations that were placed on each child. In theory, any two people raised exactly alike could end up exactly alike. I doubt this has ever been tested, and frankly, who cares? (I'm still wondering about the person who determined that no two snow flakes are alike. Can you imagine the thrill of examining billions and billions of snowflakes? All done as part of a research grant no doubt.)

When it came to persons with retardation, the box was less than empty. That person simply had less brain matter to learn or not learn. It became a vicious cycle of studying the person to see what the negative behavior really was, what caused it, and what maintained it. (The ABC's of behaviorism: antecedent, behavior, consequence.) *Staff* then determined positive or negative reinforcers for the new, more desirable, behavior. Staff would then provide the right amount of reinforcer, in the right pattern (constant, intermittent or random reinforcement). Professionals then instructed direct line staff to carry out the plan *correctly*. If the negative behavior continued, either the plan was a failure or staff failed to carry out the plan.

The wants, needs and desires of the person themselves were never considered. This was a product of the time. We knew best and therefore we didn't have to actually ask a person with a disability about their dreams ... in fact, many people didn't even believe that a person with a disability could dream! As they were successful at treating behaviors, behaviorists began to be asked to program away depression, eliminate agitation and change personality -- all things that would make a system run more smoothly. Many behaviorists said, "No!" By doing this, they suggested that a person with a disabiltiy had a right to human feelings and expressions. Some may find it odd that among the first advocates for understanding the psychiatric needs of a person with a disability were those who made the graphs, dispensed the tokens, proved that people with disabilities could learn. They were also the ones who began to suggest that their clients could feel. (Even so, we still have a long way to go. We still often negate their rights to feelings and emotions.)

As a result, such hard core beliefs are rarely evident today. Many professionals continue to use features of behavioral intervention. Let's face it, we all like to be reinforced by pats on the back, a smile, or a paycheck. Softer features have been added with the continued attempts to understand the role of antecedents, the power of reinforcers and how cognitive behavior management applies to people with disabilities. These important additions do attempt to address the needs and feelings of the person in question. Even more importantly, we are beginning to explore why the behavior exists and how the person can learn to have their needs met in a better and more appropriate manner.

The behavioral psychologists generated volumes of programs -- and we took volumes of notes. These weren't just notes, they were 'clinical records.' Trust me: some of my most useful moments will never be found in those early records. Back in the 1970's and 1980's, however, the same people on endless treatment programs which generated the notes and data were also on major tranquilizers. Although the tranquilizers assisted with the control of the aversive behavior, the interaction with the organic part of the probable psychiatric disease was not well understood. This tranquilizing effect did allow many people to be deinstitutionalized, but staff often feared 'what if?', so the medication became the long term answer for the total person, and in may instances created other organic diseases such as tardive dyskinesia.

This was a very strange time in the history of developmental disabilities. People with a developmental disability were simply not allowed to be mentally ill. Mental illness required improper parenting. It required cognition. It required abilities for insight (to their misspent youths). None of these: cognition, parents and insight were felt to be found in the developmentally disabled, previously institutionalized person. If, it was reasoned, psychiatric illness was impossible in people with developmental disabilities, then all psychiatric medications should be abandoned! Systems all over the country tried to abolish Mellaril and Thorazine (and other anti-psychotics) usage as abruptly as possible. This was disastrous for reasons we understand *now*, but not then. (See tardive withdrawal syndrome in Chapter 5). And so, the presence of the medicines -- appropriate and inappropriate continues even today.

2

All Stressed Up & Nowhere to Go

What kind of things stress you out? Have you ever been stressed out at work because you felt you had all kinds of responsibilities but no authority to make change? Do you ever feel angry when you walk in the door from a busy day at work and are informed that you need to clean the house, cut the grass and oh, yeah, the laundry needs doing? Does fear of violence ever effect you? How about concerns of whether you have enough funds to go out for some fun or for future needs? Have you ever felt like you were in a dead-end job with no chance of advancement? Have you ever lost a friend for reasons that you didn't understand?

Now if you say you never get stressed out, I can only conclude one of two things. You're six feet under, or lying. Of course, 'I am a professional.' To 'de-stress' myself, I get up at 5:30 a.m. so that I can meditate for thirty minutes, then I engage in various aerobic exercises for forty-five minutes each day. I eat only what the food pyramid allows. I *never* drink caffeine, alcohol, or anything, but pure organic juice, and spring waters. I'm also full of it.

In truth, I believe that the fact that 'stressed' spelled backwards is 'desserts' is not an accident! I have at least twenty pounds that I could stand to lose. My favorite form of exercise is lifting the flip-top of my can of Diet Pepsi (caffeinated of course).

For persons with developmental disabilities the whole picture of being 'stressed out' takes on a whole new light. A few paragraphs ago, I described some common stressors. These have all been relayed to me by various persons with disabilities. Surprised? I'm sure you were led to believe that these things only effect 'us'.

Stress can come from both inside of ourselves and from our relationship with the outside world. People with a developmental disability often suffer from many social crises. It is unfortunate, but not unusual, for persons with a developmental disability to have limited friendships. They suffer from the stigma of being disabled and are frequently looked down upon by others within a society that worships the ideal. In years past (and even today, if we are being honest with ourselves), they have been treated with many degrading approaches such as institutionalization, infantilism, and a requirement to be compliant.

Emma and I went out to lunch the other day. She is a 50 year old lady who fell out of a second story window when she was 2 years old. She had spent over 20 years in psychiatric hospitals, and currently lives in a 12 bed group home. On our way back from lunch, I was grumbling to myself about all the little chores I needed to do that afternoon. Sensing my distance, she asked what I was planning for my afternoon. I lamented briefly over my too full plans. She sighed and said, "You're lucky. You're free. You can do what you want, when you want to. I've been locked up all my life. I have to wait until someone let's me do something." Mighty profound words from someone whose case manager sat in a meeting and said that she was incapable of insight. My afternoon took on a whole new perspective. Not that I was thrilled to have to do chores, but I was grateful that I had the freedom to fill or not fill my life with all these activities.

Are you ever non-compliant? Please don't stand up and be counted, the number would be past what my calculator could reasonably expect to manage. Forced compliance is a source of major stress -- for everyone. I remember a shopping trip with a distant relative. This particular lady is well accustomed to being in charge of both herself and others around her. She's one of those people who is always impeccably groomed and in the latest of fashion. I, on the other hand, am grateful that blue jeans and cotton knit shirts, (long or short sleeve depending on the weather) are never entirely in or out of style.

On this particular shopping trip, I spotted a beautiful suit marked seventy-five percent off! If there's one thing I love more than comfortable clothes, it's a bargain. Alas, the suit was one-hundred percent wool and just touching it caused my skin to break out in an allergic rash. I put it back. My companion noticed me putting back what was probably the only potential wardrobe item she'd ever approved of. She commented "You really dress too casual." She paused then continued "And you're not going to change because I've spoken are you?" I'm not. I'm definitely a 'non-compliant' kind of person. While I didn't back down, thinking of that situation still raises my blood pressure several notches.

I was presenting a day-long conference on dual-diagnosis. A staff person was very concerned about a client he knew. He wanted to know if there was some anti-anxiety medicine that would help his client relax during her haircut. She screamed and yelled and hit others whenever it was time for a hair cut. Clearly she was non-compliant and aggressive as well. As we discussed the situation, it was noted that this non-verbal person was virtually never aggressive except at haircut time. We concluded that perhaps rather than a medication, letting her 'choose' to wear her hair long, made

15

more sense. She was being forced to comply with something she didn't like. Her only alternative was to strike out.

Although this book is unable to devote a lot of space to the area of abuse, it is an area that requires a lot of emphasis. The abuse that persons with developmental disabilities have endured at the very hands of the people hired to help them is nothing less than an abomination. There are many excellent resources regarding the nature and response of physical and/or sexual abuse in persons with disabilities. Reading most anything written by Dave Hingsburger, Dick Sobsey, or Ruth Ryan (to name a few) will provide you with far greater depth than I can hope to here. It goes without saying, however, that a population of people where huge numbers have been abused will endure -- perhaps forever -- the stress of living in environments wherein they were hurt, surrounded by people they no longer feel they can trust.

Although psychological abuse and stress do not cause psychiatric or mental illness, they can significantly weaken a physical system already over taxed from having to deal with an often confusing and complicated world. Stress can be more than just psychological. Physical illness can also be a 'stress'. I find that many people, especially those with limited verbal abilities act out physically due to pain or illness. It is tragic when this is not discovered. Recently, I read in the newspaper of a person with a disability who received over sixty punishing consequences to her behavior on the *day she died*. (Lasalandra, 1995) The problematic behavior, while recognized, was not understood to be either an indicator of the serious nature of her medical illness nor as a means of trying to wake up the professionals around her.

Ruth Ryan presented at a recent conference about the

700 plus clients her team had evaluated in Colorado. Approximately 38% have medical conditions that have significant psychiatric overlay. The people I have seen have had similar ratios of medical concerns. It is important that before an initial psychiatric consultation, and often when there is a worsening of target behaviors, that a complete evaluation of physical concerns be done to rule out any possibility of a connection. Common physical symptoms may include seizure disorders, headaches, hypothyroidism, gastro-intestinal disturbances such as gastric reflux, ulcers, milk intolerance, constipation, and/or diarrhea. Basic laboratory screenings should include chest x-ray, blood counts, liver and kidney function tests, thyroid screens, urine analysis, and others based on the individual needs of the person.

Jack rolled his wheelchair into the conference room, he was a pleasant man who seemed well liked by all who knew him. He had lived in a nursing home for over thirty years because of his cerebral palsy and 'chronic psychotic disorder.' Due to new federal guidelines, a screening process brought him to the attention of the community mental health staff. After a bit of time and a bit of preparation he moved. He loved his new group home, his new friends, and particularly his new girlfriend.

Although the community doctor continued his Mellaril 200 mg at bedtime, a prescription that he had been on for years, people were concerned that the medication was no longer working. He was becoming 'more psychotic.' Perhaps the stress of the move was too much for him. He had lost 20 pounds which was a concern as he was quite thin to begin with but what really scared the staff was his insistence that the 'wolves were howling at his door', and many nonspecific physical complaints of discomfort.

17

At first glance, Jack may have been psychotic, but some things did not fit. Most people with any type of schizophrenia (especially if the condition is worsening) have extreme difficulty with social situations. Jack loved to be with people, and people enjoyed being with him too. He looked to me like someone who simply didn't feel well (How's that for a succinct diagnosis?). He was due to see his primary care doctor again soon. We all agreed that close attention be given to the weight loss and discomfort.

Jack had cancer. Other seniors from his former nursing home had often referred to dying as 'the wolves howling at the door.' Jack is not and possibly never was psychotic. Given the type of cancer that he had, it is doubtful that even earlier intervention could have helped. What is important is to never overlook what a person is saying (verbally or non-verbally) and when we don't think that what they say makes sense, perhaps asking for an explanation might be in order!

Too, just because a person has a developmental disability, does not leave them immune to other genetically associated conditions. A question that any health provider should ask about is family history. Some of the first breakthroughs in recognizing the biochemical nature of psychiatric disorders were the 'twin studies'. In these studies, twins raised separately, together, with their biological families or adopted families were studied. It was discovered that persons with an immediate family member (especially an identical twin) with a psychiatric illness had a much higher probability of also developing a psychiatric illness. This does not condemn a person to always have an illness, but the potential is certainly higher. In this way psychiatric illnesses may be inherited a lot more like physical traits and appearances than anyone used to think.

I have a milk intolerance. If I have milk, my immediate environment is distinctly unfriendly. When I am faced with some sort of crisis, my weakened system is quickly effected. I have diarrhea. The pressing need I feel in the nether region makes it difficult to deal with anything else in my world. I stop being a competent adult, an effective decision maker, my skills as a communicator deteriorate until I'm left with only two sentences -- Get out of the way! and Get out of the bathroom --NOW! This isn't really my fault, I was born with a 'defect' in how my body operates and I am left having to avoid or cope as the situation dictates.

Using this same analogy, it goes without saying that individuals with a developmental disability often have an inherent defect somewhere within the brain. (Arnold 1993) This defect may have been a result of damage *in utero*, at the time of birth, or shortly after birth, but for some reason the brain did not develop as it should have. This provides a 'weakness' in the system such that other pathologies can occur. It comes as no surprise that seizure disorders are far more common in people with a developmental disability (twenty-one percent versus one percent of normal population Coulter, 1993).

Stress is a universal phenomenon, not just for persons with disabilities. When you are faced with stress, what do you do? Eat more? Sleep more? Talk to other people? Scream and yell? Now, if a person with a developmental disability screams and yells, that person is subject to a behavior treatment plan. We run away to the mall. They 'elope'. We go to the bar and have a drink. They engage in unhealthy life choices. We eat an extra bowl of double chocolate ice cream, they find the refrigerator locked.

I remember the day I got so angry at my husband

19

(about what, I no longer remember) that I left him with the children while I went shopping. Walking through the mall calmly looking at all the things I couldn't afford soothed me almost as much as being alone without husband and kids in tow. Oh, I know what I did was 'unhealthy.' I knew I would send hundreds of self help writers running to their typewriters. I knew that I had to deal with the whole problem when I got back home. But I also knew that I HAD to get out of there. Where I am different from a person with a disability who elopes from a stressful environment is that I had no treatment plan to face when I returned.

My best friend, unfortunately, lives another telephone area code away. Our phone bills are usually in the three digits. We have solved many of the world's crises (at least within our own worlds) on the telephone. Next to our mates, we have been each other's primary source of support. Many people with disabilities do not have somebody that they can call on the telephone who is not a relative or a paid staff. There is no one that they can just 'bitch' to about what is going on in their lives. Even if they did, they would have to wait until it is 'their night to make a phone call.'

I don't know if you have ever read the 'DD Handbook.' This is not a published book, but a hidden set of rules found in almost every agency. According to the 'DD Handbook', if you are developmentally disabled, you cannot exceed ten percent of your ideal body weight. It's a rule. One of many found in The Book. If you do exceed ten percent of your body weight, staff are going to put you on one less-than-fun diet. On Christmas Eve when everyone else is having a feast, you are going to eat carrot sticks because treatment plans know no season.

I am not diagnosed as having a disability but

someone could look at me and say, "Sue, you need to lose twenty pounds." And guess what they would find if they investigated me a little further. I have a father who has had two heart attacks. My mother also has a heart condition. WAIT! My brother has high blood pressure. Now, I'm a reasonably intelligent sort of a person. I can figure out what the odds are against me. But it's still my choice. The correct behavior treatment plan has yet to be written to change my behaviors.

I was just starting to see clients on my own. Reading through the doctor's notes I saw that Bill had low levels of aggression and was basically stable. Whew! I can handle this. I called a team meeting, some of the staff found the chairs a tad tight. They immediately start telling me how Bill's aggression level had gone through the roof. He was stealing food, non-compliant (particularly to the rule about staying out of the kitchen), and would elope to the local food store. So much for the doc's only giving me stable clients.

It turns out that shortly after his last psychiatric visit, Bill had his annual planning meeting. Middle age spread had gotten its hold on him. He was about twenty-five to thirty pounds over his ideal weight range. He was placed on a twelve-hundred calorie diet. He hated it. His 'negative' behaviors made sense to me -- he was reacting to forced compliance. The stress of living with people who felt they could just do this to him was too great for him. He was angry. What really struck me was that Bill and I were the thinnest people in the room!

Developmentally delayed? We, the experts, coined the term 'developmentally delayed'. This implies that some people require a longer time to develop. Maybe this 'delay' requires attention. Please do not interpret my line of thinking as the same as seeing a person with a disability as an 'eternal child'. What I am implying is that persons with disabilities may not have had adequate opportunities to learn coping strategies to handle their stresses. (Trust me, though, not many of my coping strategies are grown-up either.) The stress may become even greater the older the person becomes. In adulthood the stress of choosing between jobs or between possible mates (like we all had a line up to choose from) are greater than those involved in the choices we made as children. It is important that coping strategies grow along with the demands made.

Jessie (the lady from my graduate school days) was experiencing some major stressors when I first met her. She had the desire and skills to work and live more independently. Unfortunately, when challenged by stress, she reverted into typical teenage rebellion. Teenagers are at an age where they still require adult guidance and structure, but in developing their own identity they also try to break away and defy those supports.

After Jessie finished crying that very first day, I made a brilliant observation, "You look sad." She agreed. I followed that observation with a remarkable question, "Why?" She told me. Jessie's major concern was whether she could in fact continue to support herself once out of the group home. A friend of hers had 'acted bad' (had a psychotic decompensation) and was returned to the institution. She said that while she hated the institution, she knew she would always 'have a roof over my head and three meals a day.' Acting bad in order to return to the institution equalled safety for her. She understood the possible consequences of a move to a new apartment. 'If I screw up in my own apartment, I could end up a bag lady on the street.' Her aggressions and swearing must be seen as 'typical' or understandable for an 18 year old, but she has never learned how a 35 year old should cope with the stress of her first apartment.

Biochemical stresses, social stresses, abuses, and limited supports do not add up to a mentally healthy individual. For all of these reasons, eventually, it was conceded that not only could persons with a developmental disability have a psychiatric illness, but they were more likely than the average person to have a psychiatric illness (Sovner & Hurley, 1990; Eaton & Menoloseino, 1982; Reiss, S., 1982). Some estimates state the numbers may be as high as thirty percent to thirty-five percent of all clients with developmental disabilities may have an additional psychiatric impairment (Sovner & Hurley, 1990; Weber & Wimner, 1986). In fact, psychiatric impairments rank second only after mobility as an additional disability in persons with a developmental disability (Jacobson & Janicki, 1987).

If you are willing to agree that persons with developmental disabilities can have a mental illness, what does that mean? Are drugs always necessary? Mental illness is a physical illness. While a person's happiness and well-being can be affected by good and bad situations in life, mental illness has a definite physiological basis. So what's the difference between treatment of mental illness and chemical restraint?

I am not an advocate of medications in all cases. I do not receive a 'kick back' for the amount of medicines prescribed. I understand that in the past, persons with mental retardation were either over-medicated (we've all seen dazed, drugged eyes) or horribly under-medicated. People with disabilities were often routinely operated on without anesthesia! I doubt anyone reading this book today would deny any one, regardless of IQ status, the right to have anesthesia. If psychiatric medications help persons with so called normal intelligence, should they not also be available to persons with developmental disabilities? If you answer yes, then the next question is, 'in what cases should they be prescribed?'

Have you ever had a really bad cold or flu? You feel downright awful. My mom always called it feeling "Aus gescheissen" (if you're German you'll understand why I didn't translate that!). If you don't go to the doctor, it will take about four to ten days to feel better. If you do go to the doctor, you may expect some magical cure. Sometimes the patient feels so bad, they insist on a prescription for antibiotics. You will still feel better in four to ten days. Antibiotics do absolutely nothing for viruses which cause the common cold and flu. In fact, improper overuse of antibiotics has led to the creation of 'super bugs', some of which are very resistive to our current supply of antibiotics. The person is also at risk for side effects of the antibiotics. Antibiotics, however, may help avoid or cure a secondary opportunistic bacterial infection. (When a person is in a weakened condition from a cold or flu virus, other bacteria can move in and cause their own infection). Some people may swear that antibiotics are helping, but this is simply the 'placebo' effect (we feel better because we really *think* it helps, not because it does help).

Medicines used in psychiatry can have much the same effect. In many instances, a person has been placed on the 'drug of the month' hoping and praying that it helps curb negative behaviors, typically aggression and 'non-compliance'. If the person has no actual psychiatric illness, the medicine will have no effect (other than the initial

24

placebo) at best, or harmful side effects at worst. This is chemical restraint and should be avoided at all costs. On the other hand, if actual psychiatric illness does exist, it requires accurate assessment, diagnosis and treatment which may very well include *appropriate* medications in amounts that create the maximum amount of benefit with the least number of side effects.

The next few chapters will discuss the primary psychiatric categories, and their association in persons with disabilities.

3
It's the Pits

Mary came to see me today. I always look forward to our visits. Now. As usual, she started out asking about my day. After I filled her in on little bits of my life, she told me that she almost had the money saved for her next trip to Florida. Her dad, she said, was about the same in the nursing home and it is important for her to get to visit him. She worries about him being all alone. As we converse, there is that sense of shared understanding -- adult women both caring for older relatives. This is not the same Mary that I met two years ago. At our first meeting (and many after that) she arrived with disheveled hair, rumpled old clothes that were worse than necessary given her limited, but stable, income. She used to cry during the meetings. If she spoke at all, it was very slow, monotone, and always of sad topics. She always looked tired -- probably because she was. She tried to sleep, but rarely did. Mary had suffered from major depression for several years. She had a therapist that she really worked well with, but the symptoms rarely changed. Finally, she agreed to see the psychiatrist and subsequently her case was transferred to me.

Besides major depression, Mary was also diagnosed with mild mental retardation. Her symptoms had nothing to do with her intellectual functioning and everything to do with the biochemical disturbance in her brain.

Have you ever been a bean counter? The main reason I get a new referral for someone to see the psychiatrist is because the person is aggressive, either toward himself or someone else. (The latter is taken more seriously than the

Chart 3.1

Symptoms of Major Depression (DSM IV)

Must include #1 or #2, and four more symptoms:

1) Depressed mood (may appear as irritable mood)
2) Loss of interest or pleasure
3) Significant weight change when not trying to change weight
4) Insomnia or over-sleeping
5) Restlessness, or significant loss of movement
6) Fatigue, loss of energy
7) Feelings of worthlessness or excessive guilt
8) Decreased ability to concentrate, or indecisiveness
9) Recurrent thoughts of death, suicidal

former.) The team would come in to see the psychiatrist and say, "You know Doctor, George had 4.73 acts of aggression in August. In September, that number was steadily climbing to 7.38 acts of aggression, and by October, which is the last complete month that we've got of data, did you know he was up to 10.72 acts of aggression?!" People who work in developmental disabilities are good bean counters. We have been taught to count individual acts of aggression, to count individual acts of non-compliance, to count all sorts of things. After trying for a long, long time to figure out what a .38 act of aggression was, I have given up. Did the guy quit .38 seconds after starting or what? Did he hit only .38% of the intended target? Did he only hit .38% of the staff? Your guess is as good as mine.

According to Dr. Sovner (1990), persons with developmental disabilities suffer from the full range of psychiatric disorders. These disorders often present as negative behaviors. An area that is frequently over looked, but commonly present is the affective disorders or mood disorders.

According to the DSM IV, major depression has a collection of symptoms. (See Chart 3.1) Unfortunately, many health providers rely on the individual's ability to self-report. Since many persons with disabilities are non-verbal, or don't have sufficient word knowledge to describe their feelings, these disorders are often overlooked or mismanaged.

I have found the following mood scale to be helpful in gathering and following information on a person's mood. (Charts 3.2a & 3.2b). Unlike a lot of other baseline type charts that you have probably filled out somewhere, zero is not baseline for the person being monitored. The person's "baseline" may actually be a minus two on a highly regular basis.

Zero equals normal mood for anybody. (Don't look to me for a "normal" mood, but I'm told people have them!) At zero, the person smiles appropriately. They enjoy and engage in activities. They interact well with others. They sleep seven to nine hours per night without difficulty. (These are not parents by the way -- as a parent, I can testify to the effects of chronic lack of sleep.) Their appetite is stable (one Sara Lee chocolate cake instead of two?) and their concentration is appropriate to their functioning level. That's just basic mood. That's where we hope most of us sort of fit most of the time. A lot of us tend to fluctuate, between the minus one and the plus one, and that's OK. Don't go diagnosing yourself here!

Do you know anyone who has been diagnosed as clinically depressed? When I first met Mary, I used to dread our sessions. People with major depression can pull your own mood down. They're not the life of the party. If the person does talk, it's almost always of a negative subject or mood. Nothing is ever fun or good or happy. You may hear a lot of "I'm sorry," or "I'm bad." Their self-care is probably the pits.

When I work with people who are clinically, chronically depressed, sometimes I feel like smacking them up side of the head. (Remember there are no bad feelings -- they only become bad if we act on them!) I tend to feel that if they just got out more, if they just got involved in activities, if they just started talking to somebody or if they just made themselves look better they would feel better. There is that whole feeling of 'it's the person's fault'. After all we can come up with hundreds of suggestions. (All of them are the solutions we use to help us when we are previously

CHART 3.2a
THE MOOD CHART

NAME:_____   MONTH/YEAR:_____

Circle the appropriate number that corresponds
with the individual's mood/behavior for the day.
Please keep separate logs for home and school/day
activity.

+3 = severe mania   -1 = mild depression
+2 = moderate mania   -2 = moderate depression
+1 = mild mania   -3 = severe depression
  0 = normal mood

DAY

01	+3	+2	+1	0	-1	-2	-3
02	+3	+2	+1	0	-1	-2	-3
03	+3	+2	+1	0	-1	-2	-3
04	+3	+2	+1	0	-1	-2	-3
05	+3	+2	+1	0	-1	-2	-3
06	+3	+2	+1	0	-1	-2	-3
07	+3	+2	+1	0	-1	-2	-3
08	+3	+2	+1	0	-1	-2	-3
....	+3	+2	+1	0	-1	-2	-3
....	+3	+2	+1	0	-1	-2	-3
....	+3	+2	+1	0	-1	-2	-3
25	+3	+2	+1	0	-1	-2	-3
26	+3	+2	+1	0	-1	-2	-3
27	+3	+2	+1	0	-1	-2	-3
28	+3	+2	+1	0	-1	-2	-3
29	+3	+2	+1	0	-1	-2	-3
30	+3	+2	+1	0	-1	-2	-3
31	+3	+2	+1	0	-1	-2	-3

CHART 3.2b
MOOD CHART KEY

Circle the most appropriate number for the day. Pick the *larger* number when more than one item applies for the individual that day. **Note: A person is **rarely** *"very depressed"* and *"very manic"* on the same day. If moods shift this swiftly, the person is LABILE.

+3: Constant motion, frequently getting into trouble, appears unable to stop, speech is very fast and may not make its usual sense, requires less than 4-5 hours of sleep a night and does not appear tired.

+2: Extremely active, difficult to redirect, acts out without provocation and almost seems to enjoy being in trouble, eats very fast or not at all. May seem very grandiose, i.e., can do anything. Labile mood.

+1: More active, more energy than usual but not out of control. May need somewhat less sleep (i.e., 1-2 hours less). Seems more "upbeat" than would be expected. Easily distracted.

0: Smiles appropriately, enjoys and engages in activities, interacts well with others, sleeps 7-9 hours per night without difficulty, appetite is stable. Concentration appropriate to functioning level.

-1: Appears sad much of the time, does not appear to enjoy activities but will participate with encouragement. Appears tired or restless, increased or decreased desire for food.

-2: Cries frequently, will not engage in activities or conversations. Avoids people, isolates themselves. Altered sleep. Decrease in self-care skills (or does not engage in self-care even though could learn, and/or tries to prevent others from doing the self-care for them). Ability to pay attention to task at least 25% less than usual. Easily agitated, says "I'm sorry" (or equivalent) frequently.

-3: Talks of death (self and/or others'). Frequent and/or severe display of inappropriate behavior (e.g., self-injury, aggression towards others) at 25% above baseline. Does not respond to *any* successful prompts to redirect anticipated behavior.

depressed. Right? Um ... I didn't hear you.)

A hormone deficiency that most people understand is insulin dependent diabetes mellitus (IDDM). In insulin dependent diabetes, the individual's pancreas is not producing enough insulin to assist with the body's utilization of glucose (sugar). The person has to have injectable insulin to survive. People with diabetes also have to watch their diets. They have to watch their skin care. They need to take care of their eyes. Without the insulin, however, they are going to die, end of statement.

I can't "smack a diabetic up side the head" to get that pancreas producing more insulin anymore than I can smack somebody with depression up side the head and get the neurotransmitters moving in the brain.

Chart 3.3 is a highly technical schematic drawing of the nerve cells in the brain. You will notice these little buggers don't touch each other. Although the brain is responsible for relaying a major portion of information that the body needs to have, the nerve cells don't actually touch each other. The way that they communicate with one another is by a very complex system of neurotransmitters.

Although the exact mechanism of psychiatric illnesses are not entirely clear at the time of the writing (I hope in ten years this basic information is entirely obsolete), mental illness is a result of neurotransmitter failure. The illnesses are a result of either too much or too little of the transmitters being created, released, transmitted from the first cell, or received by the second cell.

It is not my purpose to detail these processes (especially since new information is now coming out rather quickly), but to provide a brief description so that there can be greater understanding of the diseases and how the medications work. For those of you with a far greater scientific understanding than myself, please forgive my simple explanations.

The neurotransmitter most commonly associated with major depression is serotonin. Quite simply, there is not enough serotonin available to the successive cells, to transmit the appropriate messages. If, *for example,* it takes one hundred serotonins to complete the signal transmission to cell #2, someone with major depression may only be providing fifty to sixty serotonins to cell #2. This creates as efficient a system as trying to run an 8 cylinder car on 5 cylinders. The car doesn't run well, if at all.

Serotonin is thought to be responsible for the regulation of mood, sleep, and to some extent appetite and 'enjoyment'. When the individual's nerve cells in the brain do not produce enough of the serotonin, the person will not feel well, regardless of that person's strength of character, moral fiber or number of smacks up the side of the head.

Let's go back to the mood scale which allows us to estimate how depressed a person might be. Let's say that Donna is at a minus one on the scale. When staff announce an outing by saying, "Come on! We're going shopping. We're going to go the mall. Joe needs underwear (won't that be an exciting shopping trip!?) Come on Donna, we're leaving." She doesn't leap up at the prospect. Staff ask a number of times, with each successive time their tone increases and their manners decrease. Finally, just because she's tired of staff bugging her, she will stand up and slowly meander her way on downstairs ready to get in the van. At the mall, she lags behind the rest of the group, but she is *not*

34

CHART 3.3

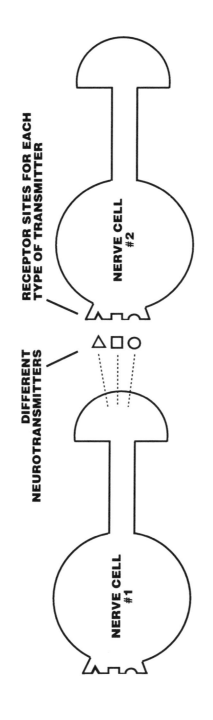

NERVE CELL #1

DIFFERENT NEUROTRANSMITTERS

RECEPTOR SITES FOR EACH TYPE OF TRANSMITTER

NERVE CELL #2

"HIGHLY TECHNICAL, TOTALLY CORRECT" DRAWING OF NERVE CELLS

having a good time. She is there, she is "complying", but she's definitely not having a good time. At the risk of agonizing over a point, enjoyment of an activity is a key concern in depression. Remember attending your significant others' high school reunion? You complied and attended. Did you *enjoy* it? Please note what the person is enjoying, not what she is supposed to be enjoying.

A person at minus one appears tired or restless much of the time. There may be some changes in sleep patterns. There is either an increased or decreased interest in food. Most typically, people who are mildly depressed will have an increased interest in food. People who are severely depressed will have a decreased interest in food. That's not universal, but that tends to be the way things go.

Let's say that Donna is now at a minus two, she cries frequently, for no apparent reason, or seemingly irrelevant reasons. She will not engage in activities that she used to enjoy or conversations. Donna tends to put herself in the corner. If Donna lives in a place where she is not allowed into her bedroom during 'program time' she will find a place to hide and here she will isolate herself. She will not participate in activities, and if you try to get her to participate in activities, she may become aggressive and you can count on this increasing during the month. Because the aggression seems linked to requests for her to participate, we may erroneously consider the aggression as a severe form of "non-compliance".

People with depression are likely to be agitated. To get a feel for this, remember the last really rotten day that you had. You have had a miserable day, anything that could have humanly gone wrong did. You got stuck in traffic on the way home. You're finally getting close to home and you remember that you were supposed to stop and pick up some bread and milk at the store. The store is ten minutes back and you're late getting to the sitter to pick up the kids. The sitter gives you that, 'one more time and you can find another sitter' look. As you walk in the house, the kids are bouncing off the ceiling because they are excited to be home. "Mom, Mom can we play a game?" "I'm hungry, can we eat right now?" and you haven't taken off your coat yet. Have you ever had that day?

Now I know none of you have ever had a bad day at work, and come home and yelled at somebody. I know that while you haven't ever done that, I have. You know that yelling at a child or spouse is irrational, but you do it anyway. The day had been more than you could handle. Freud called it displacement. I call it the "Kick the dog syndrome" (Angry at your boss? Come home and yell at the kids).

I remember standing at the check out lane with my three year old. It was long past her naptime, and mine too. We had been on the go since early in the morning. Suddenly, she spies the candy aisle. I ever so calmly explain that she hasn't had lunch yet, and this would not be a nutritionally advisable choice according to the food pyramid. (Loosely translated, I yelled 'no' because she'd already had too much junk food.) She started yelling and screaming 'out of the blue'.

It seems that when a person who is disabled becomes aggressive, or non-compliant, if we can't find an immediate source of frustration, we too assume it came 'out of the blue'. It didn't come from no where, you just may not have known what went on during that person's day. When this scenario happens at the minus two range on the depression scale, it is happening not just on the isolated bad day but all the time.

Another common symptom in depression is a sleep disturbance. Have you ever had trouble falling asleep one night? You might be very nervous about something going on the next day, and you watch the clock go by, 11:30, 12:00, 12:30, 1:00. You know you have to get up at 6:00 regardless of what time you fall asleep. You feel like screaming at that point. Staff will often report to me that Fred is up until 2:00 a.m. tearing his room apart and making so much noise, no one else can sleep. It's the same thing as your occasional night without sleep, except for the depressed person, it is a nightly occurrence. (You're thinking, "Yeah, but I don't tear the room up." See, caught you! This is true, but you work out your frustration by *thinking* about tearing the room up!) Particularly when a person is nonverbal, they act out their frustration in behavioral acts. This is much the same as those of us who are verbal. I've been told I can be pretty verbal, but even so, some days my vocabulary just doesn't serve me the way a slammed door, a banged table or a withering, hateful glance can. People with a sleep disturbance have a problem that causes frustration and requires care, it is not a function of their level of abilities nor did they plan to upset your day.

Besides trouble falling asleep, another common sleep disturbance is when people wake up frequently during the night. One of the things we ask staff or family or if possible the client themselves to do is to keep a sleep chart (Chart 3.4). Mary started by putting down what time she went to bed, what time she fell asleep, and how many times she was awake during the night. The final mark was when she woke up. We have people who will wake up frequently during the night, and stay awake longer than just going to the bathroom. Some people also wake up far earlier for work the next day, than they ever need to. They don't need to get up until 7:00 or 7:30 and they are up religiously at 5:30 in the morning ready to go. These are often symptoms of *depression*, not symptoms of irritation to the midnight shift.

Continuing on the mood scale at a minus two, as is typical with persons with depression, Mary had a decrease in self-care activities. If the depressed person cannot perform self-care for themselves, they won't allow other people to do it for them either. The staff person is in there trying to help them brush their teeth and the depressed person is smacking him out of the way. There could be two things going on here.

Number one is that people who are depressed, typically don't take care of themselves that well. Now again, some of you may not understand what I am talking about but, for me on the day when I'm not feeling particularly red hot, I don't get all dressed up. I don't bother with makeup and I lounge around in my old grubby blue jeans and old tennis shoes. Days when I'm feeling pumped up and good, I get dressed up. I put some makeup on and my good blue jeans and tennis shoes! When you are depressed, there is that feeling like you don't even deserve to look nice, because you're not worthy of it. You may even go so far as to rip up the new clothes mom just bought you.

The other thing that always needs to be taken into account, however, when somebody is particularly violent in the area of self-care, is to remember that person may have been abused. During times of self-care may have been when the abuser had free access to assault their victim. Don't forget to ask *all* the questions that need to be asked. The abuse doesn't need to be happening now for the reactions to

39

Chart 3.4

Name:_____   Month:_____

INSTRUCTIONS: Place an "A" in the box if the individual is Awake for any time during the indicated 30 minute time period. Place a "B" in the box when the person initially went to Bed, and a "U" for when he/she got Up for the next day.

DAY	1	2	3	4	5	--	--	28	29	30	31
9:00											
9:30											
10:00											
10:30											
11:00											
11:30											

18:30											
19:00											
19:30											
20:00											
20:30											
21:00											

* * Adapted from The Habilitative Healthcare Newsletter: Psych-Media Inc., PO Box 57; Bear Creek, NC 27207, c1990.

be happening now.

Before I was born, my mother tripped down a flight of stairs. She had both arms in casts. She said that the most difficult part was allowing even loved family members perform intimate self-care acts such as wiping after toiletting. After years of nursing, I am still amazed at the people who have allowed me, a stranger, to assist them with necessary activities. When I taught nursing students in a nursing home, I was never surprised when on occasion a person who had lost verbal skills acted 'aggressive'. They were saying 'no' in the only way left to them.

It's a sad but accurate reality, that many group homes have a rapid turnover of staff. When a person with multiple disabilities requires physical assistance with self-care in a group home, that person may have staff that they have never met before coming in and helping with private matters. If the person has been abused before, they won't know by a name tag if that staff can be trusted or not. The person acting violent in this scenario may or may not be depressed. One would need to look at the whole picture and react accordingly.

Also on the minus two, (still the same old mood chart) their ability to stay on task is much less than usual. When my favorite aunt passed away, no one was surprised that my work suffered for a time. I even took a leave of absence. Depressed persons are rarely able to work up to their potential. The person may express a lot of guilt -- real or imagined or say "I'm sorry" a lot. Sometimes, day program staff will say "Yeah, this guy laughs and enjoys stuff all the time." He is the first one in line when we're going on an outing to the community. He is the first one to go and grab an activity off the shelf, he's always having a good time. The

41

home staff on the other hand report something completely different. They say, "Are you kidding? We can't get him out of his bedroom." Staff in this situation were probably describing something that has more to do with his living situation and work situation than a true mental illness. In true depression the mood (or affect) will run continuous pretty much throughout that person's day, no matter where it is that they happen to find themselves.

At a minus three on the mood chart the person talks of death, either of themselves or others' a lot. Now obviously this criteria is for people who are verbal. I also want to distinguish this from those individuals who have had a relatively recent loss because then talk of death is appropriate. During the days of my aunt's funeral, people talked of other losses they have known, whether it was animals, family members, friends, or jobs. When a loss is experienced, people will bring up other losses that they are still dealing with. This is normal grieving. People who are severely depressed, however, will talk about death regardless of recent loss status.

Suicide is a primary concern in persons with depression. I have not had that many clients who have successfully committed suicide, however, for several reasons. The number one reason is that most of the people still live in such secured situations, suicide is not an option. The other thing that can happen is that for some individuals with limited cognitive abilities, they have attempted suicide, but the attempt has been something that wouldn't actually kill them. For example, taking four aspirin tablets thinking that was going to kill themselves. These folks are in the pits. They can be severely aggressive. They can be severely self-injurious. Even when they are not aggressive or self-injurious, they are not happy. They will not participate.

This is not 'non-compliance'. This is a psychiatric illness called depression. There is no behavior treatment plan that is going to get those little transmitters moving again, not even if you dole tokens out along with little smacks up the head. It's not going to happen.

The treatment options most frequently used for major depression include medications and psychotherapy. Some of the first medications used for depression are still used today. The heterocyclic (and tricyclic) anti-depressants that are still in use include Elavil and Pamelor (See Charts 3.5a&b). Although frequently effective medications, many practitioners choose not to prescribe them because of their side effect profile. The most common side effects include excessive drowsiness and constipation. For older people, there is a big problem with orthostatic hypotension. If you ever stood up too quickly and became dizzy, that's orthostatic hypotension. Other side effects can include skin reactions such as allergic rash and sun sensitivity. There are also changes in the white blood cells (infection fighters) and platelets (for blood clotting). There's more: sexual difficulties, anxiety, insomnia, increased appetite and increased risk of seizure activity. Along with these side effects is the potential risk of overdosing on these medicines for people still feeling suicidal.

Another class of medications still used are the MAO Inhibitors. Although effective in treatment of major depression, most practitioners avoid them because of their dietary restrictions. Persons taking MAO inhibitors must avoid foods high in the amino acid tyramine. Foods high in tyramine include red wine, aged cheeses, yogurt, and vinegar. The whole list is rather lengthy and restrictive in dietary choices. If these foods are eaten while on these medications, the person can experience a tyramine crisis which can cause elevated blood pressure, a stroke or even death. There must also be a two week to two month drug free period between these medications and any other antidepressant. Therefore, if these medicines don't work, there will be at least two weeks before another medicine can be tried and several more weeks before those medicines start to be effective.

Currently, the preferred drugs of choice for depression are the selective serotonin reuptake inhibitors (SSRI's). How's that for a mouth full! Nerve cells are the cells of the 90's, they recycle. When a signal needs to be transmitted from one cell to the other, cell number one spits out the correct neurotransmitter. In this case, we are talking about serotonin. After the neurotransmitters have been released out into the space between the cells, and used by the second cell, they get sucked back up by the first cell for reuse. What the SSRI's are reported to do over time is to prevent the reuptake of the serotonin, so that there is more serotonin available in this space. Over a period of time, even though cell number one only releases 50% of the necessary transmitter, there is extra serotonin available to complete the signal.

You will have noted that these medications have their effect "over a period of time". It takes any of the antidepressants 2-4 weeks, regardless of drug class, at therapeutic dosages to have their therapeutic effects but side effects can occur immediately. This is difficult at best for many people. When I take aspirin for my headache, I don't want to wait a month for it to work. I want my headache gone within 30 to 60 minutes. As annoying as my chronic sinus headaches can be, the pain involved pales compared to the pain associated with major depression. The wait is often hard, causing many people to quit and find their own more immediate reliefs, such as illicit drugs and alcohol usage or

Chart 3.5a

Antidepressant Medications

<u>Heterocyclic Antidepressants</u> - Inhibit nerve cells' ability to reabsorb norepinephrine and serotonin

amitriptyline	(Elavil)	75 mg. - 200 mg. per day [1]
amoxapine	(Asendin)	75 mg. - 200 mg. per day
desipramine	(Norpramin)	75 mg. - 200 mg. per day
imipramine	(Tofranil)	75 mg. - 200 mg. per day
nortriptyline	(Pamelor)	25 mg. - 150 mg. per day

COMMON SIDE EFFECTS INCLUDE:
Drowsiness, constipation, low blood pressure, dry mouth, urinary retention, blurry vision, confusion.

Other Possible side effects:
Allergic skin reaction, sun sensitivity (sun burn easily), changes in white blood cells and platelets, sexual difficulties including delay, inhibited, or retrograde ejaculation in males, increased anxiety or insomnia, increased appetite, risk of overdose, increased risk of seizure activity.

<u>Monoamine Oxidase Inhibitors</u> (MAOI's) - rarely used

isocarboxazid	(Marplan)	10 mg. - 50 mg. per day
phenelzine	(Nardil)	15 mg. - 75 mg. per day
tranylcypromine	(Parnate)	10 mg. - 40 mg. per day

SIDE EFFECTS RELATED TO FOOD RESTRICTIONS:
Persons on these drugs must avoid food high in Tyramine (e.g., cheese, beans, wine, pickled foods, yeast products, coffee, chocolate, soy sauce, sour cream, and many medications.

NOTE: There must be a two week (minimum) delay between taking other antidepressants and an MAOI.

---

[1] These dosage ranges are an average for most people. They can vary according to age, symptoms, response, and side effects. Some medications can be taken all at once, some several times per day.

Chart 3.5b

S.S.R.I. (Selective Serotinin Reuptake Inhibitors - Do not Significantly effect norepinephrine

fluoxetine	(Prozac)	5 mg. - 60 mg. per day
paroxetine	(Paxil)	10 mg. - 50 mg. per day
sertraline	(Zoloft)	25 mg. - 200 mg. per day
trazodone	(Desyrel)	50 mg. - 300 mg. per day
fluvoxamine	(Luvox)	50 mg. - 300 mg. per day

SIDE EFFECTS:
Trazodone and paroxetine have a sedating effect. Fluoxetine can be very activating. All can increase risk of seizures, stomach upset (especially paroxetine), delayed ejaculation in males, decreased orgasm, sweating, insomnia, anxiety, headache, diarrhea.

Other

bupropion	(Wellbutrin)	200 mg. - 450 mg. per day

SIDE EFFECTS:
Produces little or no drowsiness, effects on cardiovascular status, or weight gain. Less dry mouth, blurry vision, and confusion than heterocyclics. Greater risk of seizures.

venlafaxine	(Effexor)	75 mg. - 350 mg. per day

SIDE EFFECTS:
Major side effect is nausea/vomiting. Best taken in divided doses.

nefazodone	(Serzone)	200 mg. - 600 mg. per day

NOTE: May cause less sexual dysfunctions.

even suicide.

The side effect profiles for the SSRI's are detailed in Chart 3.5b. The most common side effect to fluoxetine (Prozac), is stimulation, much like one would feel after a strong cup of coffee. Since many depressed persons lack energy, this can be a good thing. It is advisable, however, to take it in the morning. Some people experience too much activation and cannot tolerate it. Trazodone (Desyrel) and paroxetine (Paxil), on the other hand, have a tendency towards mild sedation, and are best taken at night. Paxil is also known for causing some mild stomach upset for the first 1 to 2 weeks and is best taken with milk or food. Sertraline (Zoloft) is reported to be neither stimulatory, nor sedating. It is best absorbed, however, when taken with food. Most people take it in the morning.

Some people do not respond to the SSRI's alone. Since more than one transmitter is implicated in depression, the SSRI's alone may not provide adequate relief for all people. The heterocyclics alone or in combination with the SSRI's may be more effective. Care must be taken when adding medications together. The liver is the primary garbage disposal for ridding the body of foreign substances such as alcohol and medications. The understanding of the liver enzyme system responsible for this breakdown is in its infancy. Suffice it to say, however, that the garbage disposal can only chew up so much at any one time. Therefore, the person requiring both an SSRI and a (tri)heterocyclic antidepressant, may need less of one or both medicines. This same enzyme system is also involved with the breakdown of many medications, not just psychiatric ones. Please inform all health care providers of any medicines taken (including over-the-counter ones) because dosages of some or all of them may be affected, and some medications should not be taken together at all.

Two new medications have been released in the United States that effect the reuptake of both norepinephrine and serotonin in what scientists hope is a similar ratio actually needed by brain cells. These are Effexor (venlafaxine) and Serzone (nefazodone). Effexor is associated with a significant amount of nausea and vomiting. It is recommended that this medicine be taken two or three times per day with meals for effectiveness as well as to reduce the chance of nausea. Serzone is a cousin to trazodone (Desyrel) but is significantly less sedating.

All antidepressants can have an effect on sexuality. Most depressed people are uninterested in sex. As the depression lifts, their libido returns. Unfortunately, these medicines can commonly cause delayed ejaculation (complaints by the males, rarely their partners) in men, and sometimes inability to achieve orgasm in both men and women. Some people even say that they are not depressed, but they are dismayed with their lack of interest or response to sex. Imagine feeling better, but either feeling no sexual excitement towards your partner or being unable to experience either (or both) orgasm or ejaculation. "Gee Doc, can't I be just a little bit depressed, so I can be excited!?"

Dosages of the antidepressants can be adjusted to provide the maximal benefits with the least side effects. One medication may provide an exciting new breakthrough for those people who need long-term antidepressant therapy yet continue to have sexual problems even after dosage adjustment. Serzone is said to have specific properties to address the sexual problems unlike all the others.

People are often concerned because they have heard

that various antidepressants cause suicide. Suicide is a concern, but for an odd reason! One of the first signs that these medications are working is improved sleep patterns. When a person begins to sleep better, they begin to have more energy. Some people become so immobilized from the depression that they literally don't have the energy to attempt suicide. One to two weeks after starting these medicines can be the most critical time for suicide watch. The person has more energy, but are not yet thinking clearly, or emotionally stronger. This scenario can be true for all the antidepressants. Fortunately, not all people feel suicidal, or with close monitoring come through this period unharmed.

There are many different treatments for depression besides medications. Some centers continue to advocate for the use of electroconvulsive therapy -- ECT. For people who are so resistant to current medications, or so suicidal that time is critical, ECT may be a viable option. ECT has come a long way since its early days. At this time, persons are anesthetized then given small voltages to the brain. Literally, it is as if someone is jump starting a dead battery on a cold morning. It is believed that the seizure-like activity activates the neurotransmitters into moving again. The largest dangers to ECT include all the risks associated with anesthesia, and some persons experience amnesia about the ECT procedure, and occasionally amnesia regarding other events as well.

Also effective for mild to moderate depression, and in combination with the medications are individual and group therapy. Therapy can be helpful to assist a person deal with painful realities in their past or present life. Sometimes therapy alone is all that is necessary. If a person has not coped well with realities in their life, medications alone will never completely assist the individual. I realize that there

49

are many people who believe that persons with developmental disabilities are incapable of insight and therefore could not benefit from therapy but I assume that if you have read this far, you know better.

As with all candidates for therapy, the starting point is assessment. You need to assess what the candidate feels the problems are, what you the therapist perceives the problems to be, and (let's be real here) what the agency paying for the therapy perceives the problems to be. These three lists rarely start out the same. Somewhere in the therapeutic process, the goals may begin to blend.

As in the case of Jessie, the lady from my grad school days, she felt her primary concerns were threefold 1) I'm bad; 2) Nobody likes me; 3) I want a home of my own. From my standpoint, Jessie appeared depressed, very little self esteem, and had severely limited problem solving skills. From the agency's standpoint, she destroyed property, and was a physical threat to others in her home.

To describe the therapeutic process for individual or group therapy could be books of their own. There are more therapeutic models to choose from than the grocery store has cereals. The secret to good relationships between clients and therapists that I have seen, seems to be the respect, acceptance, and honesty that both parties bring to the relationship. The ability to speak the same language is a nice luxury to start with, but not mandatory. As people grow in a relationship, they strive to understand each other's communication patterns. People said to be "non-verbal" can also gain from a therapeutic process. Non-verbal does not mean non-communicating. Experts believe that 70% of most people's communication is non-verbal. Seventy percent is a lot to work with! Also, just because a person's mouth does not say words, does not mean she doesn't hear. In fact, it has been my experience that the more my mouth works, the less my ears do.

Group therapy can be a helpful and cost effective form of therapy. In some cases it can actually achieve more than individual therapy. One or two leaders can work with four to ten members in the same amount of time that each therapist could only see one person. Members gain support from each other. People begin to realize that others have experienced what they have. Members are often at different points of healing, such that they learn from each other.

I met Frank a few years ago. His history of abuse in the institution was rather frightening. Unfortunately, even after years in the group home where people truly cared for him, he screamed whenever he got upset. By scream, I mean that paint chips came off the walls. During one group session, Frank got upset while describing an event that had happened the previous week. Before I could react, John leaned over (John up until this point had spoken very little in the group) and said "Shut up! If you're upset, say so, but I hate your yelling!" The others agreed and asked Frank to talk instead of yell (so had staff for years, to no avail). Frank did! He later said that he never realized how his screaming bothered his friends. As staff, we were not included in that group.

Out of the Valley to the Top of the Hill

Have you ever had so much work to do that you wished you could go without sleep for a few days and not be tired? Bipolar Disorder, or manic-depression is the thing for you. The hallmark of this psychiatric illness is the ability to go for extended periods of time with little to no sleep and

51

not be tired. Now, before everyone rushes out to sign up for this illness, there are many other debilitating symptoms that go with this disorder.

Ron is the kind of guy I want with me when I have to travel to the less safe parts of town. He's big, he's strong, and he knows how to fight. Unfortunately, the way I know these things is that his fights are most often at home and in his day program. I knew Ron for over a year. Whenever I saw him, he was always on the move. He seemed to enjoy getting into trouble. He often started fights with his roommate. His roommate had had untreated depression and tried to isolate himself. Ron would deliberately provoke him. Staff said, "He acts like he is staff!" Some days he would refuse to eat, he would just keep pacing. Ron is also essentially non-verbal with the exception of nonstop sing-song utterances. He is rumored to be profoundly retarded, but no-one is sure. He wouldn't sit still long enough to be truly tested. He has been tried on Ritalin (for Attention Deficit Hyperactivity Disorder), Mellaril, and Haldol. Nothing seemed to help. At the first appointment with his new psychiatrist, staff were beside themselves. Ron had been going literally nonstop for over a week. A staff person commented that at least he knew Ron would stop soon. He was due for his 'shut down'. When asked, the staff person explained, that after an extended period of agitation, Ron always collapsed for an equal length of time where he wouldn't move. Staff were so grateful for the down times that they never told the psychiatrist about them. Ron was successfully treated for bipolar disorder. (Chart 3.6)

People with a bipolar disorder will have had forty years to complete the cycle. This is why we have a lot of people who are misdiagnosed. Suppose staff bring in a client who is acting very 'wild' (manic). If we don't have staff present that remember when he was depressed during the summer of 1992, the psychiatrist might miss the diagnosis of manic depression.

To understand mania, please look at the other half of the mood scales (Chart 3.2). At a plus one, a person is more active than usual. They have more energy, but they are not out of control. Frankly these are an enjoyable bunch of folks to have around. They may need 1 to 2 hours less sleep and they're not tired. People who are depressed are tired a lot. People who are manic are not. They seem more upbeat or agitated than you would expect. They're easily distracted. They have difficulty completing tasks because they respond to any internal or external cue that prevails.

At a plus two, the person is extremely active, they're difficult to keep on task in spite of constant supervision. They act out without provocation, and they almost seem to enjoy being in trouble. These are the people who aggravate the daylights out of staff, because they are forever getting into trouble. Unlike the depressed person off in the corner who only really gets aggressive if someone goes over and irritates them, the person with mania is right out in the middle of the room causing trouble. As a matter of fact, like Ron, they're highly likely to go over to the person in the corner and aggravate them because they know they can and they love the reaction they get.

People with mania live on the edge. It is not unusual to find out that the person is changing clothes every hour. Perhaps they begin wearing excess makeup. A person with mania may become sexually overactive and without usual precautions (unsafe sex, lacking normal discretion for partners, perhaps wanting sex with 10 different people in a day). The person may consume large quantities of alcohol or

Chart 3.6

Symptoms of a Manic Episode (DSM IV)

A. Distinct period of abnormally elevated, expansive, or irritable mood

B. During this period listed in A., the person exhibits 3 or more of the following symptoms to a significant degree:

1) Inflated self-esteem or grandiosity
2) Decreased need for sleep
3) More talkative than usual, or pressured to keep talking (may be vocalizations, not necessarily words)
4) Racing thoughts
5) Distractibility
6) Increased movements, agitation
7) Excessive pleasurable/dangerous

illicit drugs, or engage in unsafe behaviors while out in motor vehicle traffic. In short, it's like they are having a wild weekend -- all the time.

One of the complaints I hear staff say when a person is manic is 'they act like staff'. That is part of being grandiose. The opposite of feeling absolutely worthless in depression, is feeling grandiose in mania. People who are manic will believe that they are an important person of power. For many people with developmental disabilities, the perceived position of ultimate power is 'staff'.

People with mania talk fast. If you have ever listened to Robin Williams do a comic monologue, you know what manic speech is. You cannot catch everything that man says the first, second, and even third time you hear him. The man is wild and he goes from topic to topic to topic. That is exactly what manic speech sounds like. When a person is essentially non-verbal, like Ron, they may sing-song nonstop or yell almost continuously.

One thing that confuses the observer, however, is that people with mania have what is called labile moods. The person can't hold onto a mood. It is not that they are necessarily even experiencing internally all those moods as much as they can't hold onto one. The person may laugh too loud, then suddenly cry, and then immediately yell very angrily. This switch can all occur in 45 seconds. All three moods may be present in one 24 hour period. The person in not 'cycling' that fast, this is simply a variation of lability.

At a plus three, the person with mania will have unlimited amounts of energy. I have seen people with full blown mania go for over a week with out sleep and not be tired. These people can be very out of control. They can be very aggressive. The good news about somebody who is manic is that they are also very distractable. Betty could be getting ready to punch the daylights out of George when I can call and say, "Hey Betty, come on and take a look at this thing over here." Betty would probably just walk away and forget what it was she was even going to do to George. The problem then becomes George, who doesn't forget and you really need someone to help him calm down! Persons with mania *cannot* sit down to eat at the average group home table. You may only be able to get them to eat 'finger foods' and beverages as they walk by. Trying to get him to sit down to eat is inviting an act of aggression.

To experience mania, the closest I can relate this to, is a children's oriented pizza parlor that I occasionally break down and take my kids to. To start with, it's mandatory to go there on a rainy Saturday afternoon. In one corner, they have a *bazillion* and one tables and huge mechanical robots that sing these stupid songs about four decibels louder than anybody ever needs to hear them. In another corner they have video arcade games and skee ball games with wooden balls (that's a wonderful thing to give small children who are hyped up -- wooden balls). All this game playing is in pursuit of tickets so that they can get a plastic toy that's going to get lost in the car on the way home. In another corner, they have little mechanical rides that go up and down, side to side and back and forth so that the kids can puke because we just fed them all kinds of birthday cake, pizza and red dye. Usually, there are fourteen birthday parties going on with at least eight children minimum per party and all the kids are screaming.

Now the place you want to stand is near the bathroom door. Find something to do to keep busy and you will see grandparents fight each other saying, "No, it's my turn to take her to the bathroom!" The stimuli is so overwhelming that people will do almost anything to get out of it. I was giving this same example at an ARC conference and one of the women raised her hand and said, "You know, I used to work there and we used to fight each other over who got to clean the toilets." Now, I don't know about you, but I find it a sad state of affairs when you're fighting someone else for an opportunity to clean a toilet. It's plain sensory overload to the worst degree.

For a person who is manic, living in the average group home, or attending day program is like that pizza parlor on a rainy Saturday afternoon. Even as you read this book, you are giving attention to the words and tuning out many other stimuli. The kids could be yelling, or if you are at work, the boss could be yelling. You may be getting so bored that your eyes are itching, the chair may be hard, or the lighting harsh. For the most part, however, the average person is able to tune out all extraneous stuff, both internal and external. A person who is manic cannot do that. They cannot filter out stimuli and so the observer sees wild, scattered, distractable, behavior.

Just like the grandparents fighting in the pizza place, I have seen people with mania, deliberately start a fight just to get to the 'time out room'. Sometimes, when a person recognizes that they are stressed out, they are not allowed the normal releases that you and I enjoy. (Call a co-worker on the phone, go outside for a smoke, go to the restroom, grab your 5th cup of coffee for the day, wander to the photocopier machine.) Rather than use a quiet corner as punishment, better to use it as a reward. Let the person go and calm down *before* she hits someone. This is therapy, not punishment!

The actual nervous system deficits involved with bipolar disorder are still to a great extent uncertain. Consquently, although we have several medications that work to treat bipolar disorder, no one is entirely certain how they work. Lithium has been the number one drug of choice for most people with bipolar disorder for a long time. It's a naturally occurring salt found in nature It is commonly abbreviated $LiCO_3$. The other two medications that are often used are Valproic Acid (Depakote) and Carbamazapine (Tegretol).

Many people will remember that practitioners would try a person who was aggressive on Tegretol saying, "For some people, Tegretol stops the aggression, and for some it doesn't. We'll try it and see." The reason Tegretol worked in many of these cases was that both Tegretol and Depakote are effective in treating bipolar disorder. Therefore, with someone who was aggressive as a result of mood instability, Tegretol and Depakote worked.

Earlier, it was mentioned that people with developmental disabilities have a higher than average chance of also having a seizure disorder. Since Depakote and Tegretol are primarily used for seizures, it is optimal to work with the neurologist to see if either Tegretol or Depakote would work for their seizure disorder as well.

Just as an aside, research is showing that phenobarbital and Mysoline may cause aggression all on their own without other psychiatric symptomatology. My first recommendation when a person is aggressive and on one or both of those medications, is to request that the prescribing doctor consider changing to a different seizure medication. In every person that I have seen switched, all of them had a marked decrease in aggression.

Joann is a wonderful woman who lives in her own home with supports. Her supporters clearly love her, but they are worn out. Joann is always on the go. She is busy all the time, but has trouble finishing anything. She talks nonstop. Staff wondered if she had some type of anxiety disorder. Although she might, when anti-anxiety medicines were given for dental appointments, she seemed to get worse. The neighbors were complaining that Joann was up all hours of the night. She never seemed tired. The only other medicine that Joann was on was Depakote for her seizure disorder.

As you can see from Chart 3.7, the normal blood range for Depakote is 50-100 mcg/ml. Joann's blood level was 50-55. Since she had been seizure free for years, no one saw any need to increase her dosage. I met with her primary care doctor who was prescribing the Depakote. The doctor wanted to help with Joann's more difficult behaviors, but wasn't sure how. Given the lack of need for sleep, constant activity, and talking, a preliminary diagnosis of bipolar disorder seemed appropriate. As she was already on Depakote, the easiest move was to increase it for bipolar disorder, without hurting the seizure disorder. The last I heard, people commented that she comes home from work tired like everyone else, and really seems to be enjoying her life even more. Even the neighbors are reported to be resting better!

Depakote, Tegretol and Lithium are all blood level dependent not dose dependent. That means, for a person to achieve maximum helpful effects without harmful toxic effects, simple blood tests must be performed. The blood value has to be correlated to the person's clinical picture. One person may only need Lithium 300mg. at night to obtain a blood level of 0.6, and be relatively symptom free.

Chart 3.7

Medications for use in Bipolar Disorder
(Manic - Depression)

	Desired Blood Range[1]	Toxic Levels
carbamazepine (Tegretol)	4 - 12 mcg/ml	Greater than 15
lithium carbonate (Lithium, Eskalith)	0.5 - 1.2 mEq/liter	Greater than 2.0
valproic acid (Depakote, Depakene)	50 - 100 mcg/ml	Greater than 150

Other Drugs Used For Mania

clonazepam (Klonopin) clonidine (Catapres)	1.5- 20 mg. per day (normal dosage range)

---

[1] Actual milligrams or number of pills taken per day will vary with each person. Blood levels should be drawn 5 to 10 days after a dosage change or at least every three months, along with other relevent blood tests.

The next person may require 600mg. three times a day to obtain a blood level of 0.6, and is still experiencing symptoms. Some people with bipolar disorder do not respond well to any one of the medications alone and may require a combination of two out of the three choices.

Side effects of these three medications and toxic effects of these medications are not the same. Side effects most frequently occur when the medicines are begun or increased. All of these medicines can cause slowing of mental processes and caution should be used when starting any medication. A decision must be made on whether the disorder being treated or the side effects of the treatment are the most harmful to the person.

Toxic effects of these medications literally look as if that individual were drunk. The person may experience an irregular gait. The person may be very difficult to arouse. His speech may become very, very garbled. He may complain of feeling really lousy like he has a hangover. Another lesson in "Sue's DD Handbook": a person will only become toxic on these medications on a Friday evening before a holiday weekend, when nobody can be reached. On Tuesday morning when everybody can be reached, no one will ever become toxic.

Any person who is associated with a person on seizure medications or Lithium, should always be aware of the person acting very tired, stumbling, slurred speech, or difficult to arouse. DO NOT give the next dosage of medication. You can do more harm by giving it than by withholding it when a person is not toxic. The person will need an emergency blood draw at their usual laboratory or at the closest emergency room. When the person is toxic, medication will probably be held for a few days then gradually resumed. When the blood levels for these medications reach toxic levels, they can cause very serious damage to the liver and/or the kidneys, even to a point where they can kill.

What kinds of events can make a person toxic? Good question. I'm glad you asked that. First of all, Lithium is a salt. It will make people thirstier. Table salt is generally not restricted for a person taking Lithium. If a fluid restriction is necessary, for other reasons, the person should be carefully monitored. Generally, it doesn't matter how much liquid a person usually drinks per day (a little or a lot), as long as the amounts stay reasonably constant each day.

Toxicity occurs when the concentration levels of the drugs increase in the body. If a person has diarrhea, or is vomiting, or sweating excessively, the person is at risk for dehydration. As the internal fluid levels in the body decrease, the percentage amount of the medication in the blood increases. A person with a flu virus, for example, is in danger of becoming toxic. If a person is placed on a diuretic ("water pill"), while on these medicines, they could become toxic very quickly.

Whenever a person is on these medications (or any medications for that matter), all health providers must be notified. For example, Tegretal causes the liver to be activated such that the liver metabolizes Tegretal and other medications quicker. Women taking oral contraceptives could become pregnant if they are also taking Tegretal. Other medications, given at the same time may cause an increase in drug levels of these medications.

Before starting any of these medications, the person must undergo some basic preliminary health screenings. The person should have had a thorough physical recently. Initial lab tests should include a complete blood count, liver and kidney function tests, a urine analysis, and for Lithium an annual TSH, and EKG is recommended for anyone over the age of 40. Blood levels and appropriate other screenings should be done 5-10 days after each dosage change. When the person has reached a satisfactory blood level and is psychiatrically stable, blood levels should be drawn as well as liver and kidney function tests for Depakote, or a complete blood count for Tegretol every 3 months and full laboratory tests yearly. The blood levels of the medicines are generally drawn 10-12 hours after the last dosage. Usually the morning dose is held until the blood is taken. If the blood is taken soon after the medicine is given, it will give a falsely high level.

When I first met Terry, she reminded me of some wild untamed creature. She screamed almost nonstop. She appeared to deliberately fall if given the chance. She assaulted people violently. She had few apparent skills, and no friends.

The last time I saw her, we looked through books together. She had recently had her hair done. I am told that she informed the stylist that she was not satisfied with the first style, and for the stylist to try again. She looked very sharp. I had been covering for her primary psychiatrist who was out on leave. She asked me where her doctor was. You must understand that Terry is said to be profoundly retarded, and until recently, few of us knew she could talk. Before I could explain where the doctor was, staff interrupted and tried to tell Terry that I was the doctor. Terry very slowly explained to them (so that hopefully they would understand with only one explanation!) that "No! That's Sue. Where's the doctor?"

Terry's psychiatrist (the one on leave) had been slowly reducing the Mellaril, and placed her on Depakote. The Depakote is controlling the mania that she probably suffered from for years. The removal of the clouding effects of the antipsychotic is allowing her wonderful personality complete with wonderful sense of humor to emerge.

4
Anxiety Disorders
(Adrenaline Levels Ready for Take-off)

Annie is a thirty year old female diagnosed with Rubella Syndrome. People with rubella syndrome have many challenges to face beside having a developmental disability. The syndrome leaves people also dealing with blindness and deafness. Her communication then is essentially non-verbal. After an in-service on dual diagnosis that I had given, Annie's staff recognized the symptoms of anxiety in this lady (an occupational hazard!) and asked me to meet her. Gladly. When we met, Annie certainly looked anxious. She continuously rocked back and forth, she crossed her legs repeatedly. She rubbed her hands together almost nonstop. The look on her face was worse than my husband's just before we were married.

As my own mind raced frantically to figure out how to help this distressed team (Ativan for the team?), I stopped to look at this meeting from Annie's perspective. She hadn't seemed nervous until I actually entered the room. How had she known I was there? It is amazing that some people feel that if you can't see and hear that you have lost all your senses. This is not true! She recognized me by smell, of course. She identifies familiar people by their smell. I went over to her chair and gave her my hand. Sure enough, she smelled it, and slowly relaxed.

I tried to picture what staff were doing to help her from her perspective as the 'helpee'. Staff had been attempting to increase her sensory input by trying to expose her to a variety of new situations. Annie could not

65

determine real dangers such as walls and curbs when in unfamiliar territory. This is when she became most anxious. Once we all viewed this situation from her standpoint, changes in her programming were made that reflected this new understanding, that 'new situations' were 'scary situations.'

Annie had also been on multiple treatment plans for head banging behaviors. As part of the investigation she was given a full medical. Thank heavens! The head banging was actually Annie's non-verbal attempt to tell staff that she had sinus headaches. Once this had been diagnosed and sinus headache medicine administered at the onset of head banging, this 'negative behavior' stopped entirely.

Annie was a prime example of someone who had a legitimate psychiatric disorder (generalized anxiety disorder), but responded exceedingly well to interventions other than medication. Like depression, many of the anxiety disorders respond well to environmental changes, and other therapeutic modes such as counselling as well as behavioral approaches. Some people are assisted by medication alone. Others need therapeutic supports, but only respond to individual or group therapy after the medication has helped.

If you are from a climate that has snow and ice every winter, you will be able to understand the next scenario. For those of you from warmer climes, humor us and pretend you can relate -- remember having empathy for someone does not require you to have experienced the same situation. Have you ever skidded out on a patch of ice in your car? OK, good. What did you feel like afterwards? Helpless, rapid heart beat, wobbly legs, shaky hands, sweat stains down to the floor? You may have had to park and get out of your car because you felt out of control. You may even have had a reaction as serious as upset stomach or diarrhea.

That, my friend, is anxiety. That's exactly what anxiety feels like. Anxiety is an adrenaline rush that is out of control. Your adrenal glands are these little things that sit on top of your kidneys. Back in the age of the dinosaurs, Og had to take a look at the dinosaur and decide to run like heck or kill supper. The 'fight or flight' syndrome, if you will. Adrenaline gave Og the energy to run or fight. Adrenaline continues to do this for us today. Fortunately, we don't have actual dinosaurs to contend with, but all of us face stress in our lives. (And an occasional boss that looks a bit like a T Rex -- with PMS!) When faced with stress, our bodies react by releasing adrenaline to help us cope. We have the extra energy to fight or flee our stress.

If the smoke alarms went off while you were reading this book, and you just sat there, that wouldn't be a healthy choice. No, you would most likely get a sudden surge of energy to help you run from the building. Some of you might even panic and race off in the wrong direction because the adrenaline rush was so severe that you could not function and all you knew was to run. (Thinking and running, now that's a better option, I'd like to actually accomplish that sometime!)

Some of us never seem to get our paper work done ahead of time. The standard reason we wait until the last minutes is, "I work best under pressure!" It is true that a little bit of pressure provides a little bit of adrenaline that allows you to get things done. Without it, we would all be blobs on the couch. However, when that system goes haywire, we have anxiety disorders.

The anxiety disorders are probably the second largest

type of psychiatric disorders. For people with disabilities, this is primarily because of the issues of trauma that we are now recognizing in peoples' lives (physical abuse, sexual abuse, emotional abuse and neglect). There are many other theories for the origin of anxiety disorders. It could have been some sort of mis-configuration or structural defect in the brain, such that the chemicals that go down to the adrenal glands telling them to shoot out the adrenaline are screwed up. It could be that your body is over sensitive to even normal amounts of adrenaline that cruise through your blood vessels and react on various body organs. The theories behind anxiety disorders are as varied as those for the other disorders. Since there are different types of anxiety problems, it makes sense that there are more than one cause, and more than one treatment.

In generalized anxiety disorder (GAD), (Chart 4.1) the person is on hyper alert at all times. These people know where everybody in the environment is. They're the ones who stand in the corner, but unlike the depressed person who's got their back turned to avoid everyone, the person with GAD has their back to the corner so that they can watch and know where everybody is at any and all times. They experience many of the symptoms of anxiety much like the driver who hits the ice and skids. Since many of these symptoms are physical, people often see many medical doctors before identifying the anxiety disorder. It is important, however, to rule out medical disorders FIRST before assuming the person has a GAD. The person may also have an anxiety disorder AND other medical complications such as high blood pressure and ulcers as a result of long term anxiety.

Another of the anxiety disorders is Obsessive Compulsion Disorder (OCD) (Chart 4.2). One fellow I worked with, Dave, told me I could recount his story, he's very proud of his progress. A few years ago, a case manager of a group home asked me casually if chlomipramine (Anafranil) could cause constipation. Thinking it was only a simple question I answered, "Yes." I was about to leave until I noticed the look on her face. Then she said, "I'm not sure I should mention this..?" I always love those opening lines.

She went on to say that Dave had been very constipated lately. How constipated? "Well...Last weekend we gave him some magnesium citrate." Mag Citrate is that stuff that they try and convince you tastes like soda pop. It doesn't. One bottle, however, is usually enough to clean the average person out for intestinal X-rays. "SIX!!?" It took that much to unplug him. He was miserable. Staff didn't realize the medicine was constipating, and never knew to share that information with his doctor.

Dave has Down Syndrome. He had been labelled 'non-compliant' for years. It was his violence that caused his home staff to approach the psychiatrist. He became very violent if anyone sat in 'his' chair. In fact, if anyone sat in a seat other then their usual chair, Dave became violent. He could only leave his day program at 3:00. If he had an appointment, or the van was late, he threw things. He was so insistent on sameness that he never seemed to enjoy anything. He rarely spoke. He certainly didn't smile.

The psychiatrist determined that his non-compliance was actually Obsessive Compulsive Disorder (OCD). Although the Anafranil helped, he still had problems. Attempts to increase his medicine, resulted in the now realized constipation. Dave's team asked if anything could

Chart 4.1

Symptoms of Generalized Anxiety Disorder [GAD] (DSM IV)

A.   Excessive anxiety and worry lasting more than six months

B.   Person finds it difficult to control the worry

C.   Anxiety and worry associated with at least 3 of the following:

      1)   Restlessness, keyed up, or "on edge"

      2)   Easily fatigued

      3)   Difficulty concentrating, mind goes blank

      4)   Irritability

      5)   Muscle tension

      6)   Sleep disturbences

Other Anxiety Disorders Found in Persons with Disabilities:
- Panic Attacks
- Agoraphobia (fear of public places)
- Social phobia (fear of social situations)

Chart 4.2

Symptoms of Obsessive - Compulsive Disorder [OCD] (DSM IV)

A. Either obsessions or compulsions (may have both)

Obsessions:

1) Recurrent, persistent thoughts that are intrusive, inappropriate, and cause marked anxiety or distress
2) Thoughts suggested in #1 are not worries about real-life problems
3) Person attempts to ignore, suppress thoughts, or to neutralize them with other thoughts or actions
4) Person recognizes thoughts are of his own making

Compulsions:

1) Repetitive behaviors in response to obsession, or according to rigidly held rules
2) Behaviors are aimed at reducing or preventing distress

Also: Obsessions or Compulsions take up more than 1 hour per day, or significantly impair social, relational, or occupational functioning.

be done. Fortunately, fluoxentine (Prozac) was also found to help with compulsive behaviors. The switch was made.

At our last meeting, Dave left work early to be there. He sat in a staff person's usual chair, and laughed when the staff person mildly complained. He told several good jokes. He is now described as a 'laid back, take it as it comes' kind of guy. Violence is a thing of the past.

Obsessive Compulsive Disorder (Chart 4.2) can be an incredibly debilitating disorder. Besides the DSM IV, another very useful screening device is the "Compulsive Behaviour Checklist" designed for persons with developmental disabilities. (Gedye, 1992). Some people experience recurring thoughts that they know are of their own making. They know the ideas, images and fears are not real. In spite of this, they cannot stop the thoughts, in effect, they can start them but not stop them. Often the thoughts are of a perceived unpleasant subject such as noxious sexual activities, dislikes for another person or activity. Some people attempt to deal with these thoughts through repetitive actions such as washing their hands 23 times before eating. Some people insist on absolute sameness in routines, staff, and activities, such that any change in routine is felt to be catastrophic.

Shirley had difficulty with 'deliberate incontinence'. She could never get to the bathroom on time although repeated medical tests could reveal nothing. Closer examination showed that the kitchen was between her and the bathroom. Before she could get to the bathroom, she had to straighten up the soap dish, and make sure the cupboards doors were all closed. She had to make sure that the trash can was at the right angle. She had to make sure that the washcloth was hanging over the sink in the proper spot. By the time she finished and checked it four times, she hadn't made it to the bathroom and would have a toileting accident.

Jim went to see his general practitioner, he has high blood pressure (which is not a surprise for people with anxiety disorders). The doctor had taken his blood pressure and put the blood pressure cuff away in the top drawer. Time went on and about three months later the doctor rechecked his blood pressure. After the doctor took Jim's blood pressure, he put the cuff back in a different drawer. Jim leapt off the examining table, grabbed the blood pressure cuff, and put it back where it had been placed the first time three months ago. He too was described as aggressive and non-compliant. Dave, Shirley and Jim were helped with medications. After the medications were begun, they were all able to learn new ways of dealing with stress and enjoy life.

People with OCD attempt to control their feelings of being 'out of control' by insisting on sameness. If anything changes, the anxiety goes out of control, and thus they are out of control. Some people with OCD attempt to maintain personal control by constantly arranging things and checking them. When other people attempt to stop them from arranging, or make changes, the person with OCD may respond by attacking themselves or the changer. 'The Changer' is seen as interrupting the only way that they know to cope. Their aggression while regrettable is under-standable. If you knew, absolutely knew, that washing your hands would save you from catastrophic illness, what would you do to someone who tried to stop you? The answer lies in helping the person find better ways to cope with stress. Here the answer lies only partly with the medication and partly by teaching them new ways to control their reactions to the environment.

Many people with OCD can be assisted to control their impulses with behavioral techniques. Medications can also be a valuable tool in the treatment of OCD. The most common medications used for the treatment of OCD include chlomipramine (Anafranil), fluoxetine (Prozac), sertaline (Zoloft), and paroxatine (Paxil). Another SSRI has been used in Canada for many years for both Depression and OCD. Luvox (Fluvoxatine) has been recently released in the United States for OCD alone. Although officially classified as antidepressants, the SSRI's as a group have been shown to be very effective in all the anxiety disorders. The exact mechanisms of brain neurotransmission of serotonin and of their effect on anxiety are uncertain, but researchers do see a connection. In fact, there is a very high number of people with anxiety disorders who are also depressed. (Or is that depressed and also anxious!?) The medications have also been shown effective for the ritualistic behaviors associated with autism.

Post traumatic stress disorder (PTSD) is becoming one of the most prevalent disorders in dual diagnosis. The reason for this is simple. Persons with developmental disabilities have been subjected to incredible amounts of abuse and neglect. Some experts estimate the percentage of physical or sexual abuse in adult men who have been institutionalized to be 60%! The estimates for institutionalized women is even higher at 80%!!

Dr. Ruth Ryan (1993) found that approximately 16% of persons with a history of abuse to also have PTSD. The simple math says that over 10% of institutionalized adults are scarred by abuse that will show itself in one way or another. Often problem behaviors go uninvestigated and without the diagnosis of PTSD a treatment plan will only continue to bury the scars under layers of compliance programming. What is Post Traumatic Stress Disorder? Perhaps you can recall something that happened five or ten years ago that was a fairly traumatic situation in your life: loss of a job, loss of a loved one, or the break up of a friendship. You can look back five, ten years later and remember the unpleasantness. But frankly, if you think about it now, for the most part you realize that life went on. You've met new people, have a different job, you may even realize that you can't quite remember what all the fuss was about.

In Post Traumatic Stress Disorder, the individual experiences events that are above and beyond the ordinary. These events would be traumatic to anyone. The person remains severely traumatized even years later and the intensity of the feelings do not diminish over time. For some people, the event was so traumatic that they couldn't deal with it at the time. They bury the memories. But then something happens that begins to re-trigger the events, and once the walls that kept the memories under control start crashing down, there is no putting them back up. People may have flashbacks or nightmares about the trauma. A triggering event might be seeing a child at the same age they were at a time of the abusive situation. The person might hear about something that sounds similar to their situation.

For one young lady I was working with, the triggering event was her biological father attempting to see her one Christmas. Sara lives in an AFC home. She had graduated from school and had a job working as a grocery stocker. Her case manager was concerned because all of a sudden she was in danger of losing her job because she was stealing and binging on food.

I asked if she had any history of abuse and no one was certain. I went back to the file which, blessedly for me, was only 2 inches thick. In the file was a report from years ago when she was about ten years of age. This was when she was made a permanent ward of the state, she had been subjected to repeated abuse by her biological father, her biological mother, 'Uncles' Fred, Tom, Harry and anybody else that came along. Some of the stories in this report were nauseating. Her father's phone call started bringing the walls down. The binging was a result all of the anxiety from the sudden flood of memories.

Dr. Ryan (1993) recommends a six point protocol for treatment of PTSD. It is presumed that this protocol would also be useful for those persons who have a history of abuse, but without diagnosable PTSD. (Some people may not meet the full criteria for PTSD, but continue to have difficulties after the abusive situation that were not present before the abuse.) The protocol includes:

1) careful use of appropriate medications, but NOT just medications alone.
2) a complete medical evaluation and treatment of any additional health concerns.
3) reduce complications of other medication or treatments (i.e. side effects from other medicines, insisting the person eat foods forced on them by the abuser because it's good for them)
4) individual and/or group therapy.
5) change situations in the environment to avoid triggering events. Some persons are still forced to visit abusing family members. A person who is sent to their room as punishment may trigger memories of being locked up in isolation.
6) lots of staff and family training and support. Front line staff are unfortunately some of the last ones to

learn about PTSD and the first ones to be assaulted when they inadvertently trigger a memory.

Please note, unless the entire protocol is put into action, successful treatment will not happen. A person cannot simply be medicated and expected to improve. I have also witnessed cases where the individual was given 'therapy' and then sent back to the abusive situation. Obviously, this person got worse instead of better. In this case, the 'therapist' knew of the abuse, and still sent the person back into the abusive home. The abused person learned to trust no one.

Sometimes, people are given short-acting antianxiety medicines to help them with medical procedures. I sometimes wonder, however, if we aren't further traumatizing people, by reducing their abilities to fight frightening situations. Now let's face it, if you have been sexually abused, a gynaecological appointment is not a fun time. We should not wonder why a person who is non-verbal screams, screeches and goes racing out of the room when the doctor tries to get a pap smear. Some innovative programs are now recognizing these factors and will take as many appointments as necessary to help a person with their fears before doing the pap smear. When such programs are not available, consideration must be given on what is more important -- the fright of the test, or the potential risks of not doing the test. There are no universal answers for this.

Although I wish I didn't need to add this, I will. All people will recognize abuse regardless of someone else's determination of their IQ or abilities. I add this because I was describing symptoms of PTSD found in a woman said to be profoundly retarded. The person I was talking with, stopped me and asked "How would someone like that even know they had been abused?" This is a misconception that assumes that simply because a person scores low on arbitrary intelligence tests, they have no feelings, no memories, or more accurately stated, no heart, no mind. Besides believing that some people with disabilities cannot feel, there is the misconception that no one would find 'someone like that' physically attractive. Therefore, they would never be sexually loved so if they are violated, 'someone like that' should be grateful. Finally, rape is about abuse, control and violence not sex. The abuser most typically prefers a victim that has trouble communicating, or at least that others will not believe.

I was recently asked to provide therapy for a young woman who had been sexually abused for years by a neighbor. The neighbor was not prosecuted and sent to prison when my client's abuse was discovered. He did not go to prison until he had abused 'a normal' person. This is outrageous for two reasons. First, my client was not believed and not allowed the opportunity to press charges in court because of her disability. Second, the second young woman would never have been abused if the abuser had been tried and convicted the first time!

Barbara is 72 years old. During our initial assessment, a review of the files indicated that all of her major decompensations happened on or just before a certain date. Nothing useful was in the file to indicate what had happened. I asked Barbara. She screamed that July was a terrible month, and left the room.

In spite of staff's best efforts, come July, she had a major decompensation and had to be hospitalized. While there, she began talking about the baby. Ultimately, it was discovered that she had been raped, and impregnated.

When the baby was born, she was told that the baby was dead, and she never got to hold it. The baby's birthday was in July. She had never forgotten. Because she was 'slow', and said to be psychotic, all her talk of babies and danger was disregarded as delusional.

One fine autumn morning last year, staff gathered to plant a garden in memory of the baby. Barbara could not handle the situation and refused to attend. She gave staff permission to proceed with the planting, however. This spring, the flowers came up. July came and went and Barbara is doing better.

Prior to her last hospitalization, when Barbara screamed or became violent, the treatment plan indicated 'time out' as the best option. She was sent to a room to stay by herself until she calmed down. After finding out more about her, staff asked her what would help when she had a flashback. Barbara asked staff to hold her hand and stay by her until her fears went away. They are, they do.

Besides the SSRI's discussed earlier, there are many other anti-anxiety medications on the market. Medications called beta-blockers are usually used to treat high blood pressure. These medications include propranolol (Inderal), nadolol (Corgard) and metaprolol (Lopressor). Beta-blockers work particularly well in the "performance" anxiety disorders, that is, social phobias, fear of public places and public events. They appear to work by blocking the body's response to the adrenaline in the blood stream. The beta-blockers have also been used for treatment of rage behaviors, and treatment resistant bipolar disorder.

It is strongly recommended to have the person evaluated by their primary care doctor before initiating beta-blockers due to their effects on the circulatory system. Persons receiving these medications should have their pulse and blood pressure monitored regularly (no less than weekly). The drugs should be withheld if the pulse rate goes below 60 beats/minute, or if the blood pressure goes below 90/60. Another concern is that a side effect of the beta-blockers is depression. Other side effects include dizziness (especially if the person stands too fast), cold hands and feet, and occasionally, confusion. If the cold hands and feet are severe, or if the person appears confused, contact your doctor immediately. DO NOT ACT ON YOUR OWN. These medicines should not be stopped suddenly unless directed by your doctor.

Although most anti-anxiety medications are marketed to only be used on a short term basis, many are prescribed to the general public for years at a time. Some of these medications can be abused because of their often addictive potential. That said, the anxiolytics can still be useful for the treatment of anxiety disorders when properly prescribed.

The benzodiazepines as a group have been used for anxiety disorders and occasionally seizure disorders for years. Some people are concerned that these medications can cause physical addiction. While that is true, few of my clients are in a position to find illegal sources of the medicines to feed their habits. All physical addiction means in this case is that the medications cannot be stopped abruptly. The gradual weaning process will take time, but not near as long as it does from the anti-psychotics.

Most of the anti-anxiety medications can cause drowsiness, and the benzodiazepines are no exception. Persons taking these medicines may have trouble concentrating especially initially. The biggest concern for the benzodiazepines as a group in persons with disabilities, however, is their tendency to disinhibit some people. All people have occasional inclinations to act in 'socially unacceptable ways.' That is, they hurt others or hurt themselves, they swear, or they may publicly display private body parts, or in general act like students on spring break in Florida! Most people have internal controls that prevent them from engaging in these behaviors. This group of medications (the benzodiazepines) can eliminate those normal controls. This is called disinhibition. It is always important to report how any and all medications have effected an individual when talking with health providers.

Most clinicians have preferences for usage and avoidance of various medications. My personal bias is to not use the very short acting medications on a regular basis. They get into the system and out of the system fairly quickly. If someone has a chronic anxiety disorder, where they are feeling anxious all the time, and I prescribe a very short acting mediation, it may put them on a merry-go-round. They take a pill, and feel better for a few hours, but then they start feeling worse again. They take another dose, and they start feeling better for a few hours, but then they feel worse again. In these instances, a better option may be the longer acting anti-anxiety medication such as clonazepam (Klonopin).

Wide scale abuse of the benzodiazepines has caused clinicians to seek safer long-term anti-anxiety medications. There is a large overlap of people who have an anxiety disorder, and also have depression. When the SSRI's were first used in persons with depression it was noticed that they felt less depressed *and* less anxious! A new era of treatment had begun. Unfortunately, as stated in Chapter 3, the SSRI's and another anti-anxiety medication buspirone

Chart 4.3

Antianxiety Medications

Generic/Brand Name	Short/ Long Acting	Potential for Addiction	Drowsiness and Decreased Concentration	Cautions	Other Uses
alprazolam (Xanax)	short	yes	yes	potential for disinhibition	
buspirone (Buspar)	long	no	no	few reported side effects	anxiety associated with autism disorders
chlordiazepoxide (Librium)	short	yes	yes	potential for disinhibition	alcohol detoxification
clomipramine (Anafranil)	long	no	yes	very constipating	OCD, depression

diazepam (Valium)	long	yes	yes	potential for disinhibition	seizures, status epilepticus
clonazepam (Klonopin)	long	yes	yes	potential for disinhibition	seizures, mania
lorazepam (Ativan)	short	yes	yes	potential for disinhibition	
oxazepam (Serax)	long	yes	yes	potential for disinhibition	
clorazepate (Tranxene)	long	yes	yes	potential for disinhibition	

Other antianxiety medications:
  beta blockers used for treatment of high blood pressure, SSRI's

CANADA - All are benzodiazepams
  clobazam (Frisium)
  ketazolam (Loftran)
  nitrazepam (Mogadon)

(Buspar) take several weeks at therapeutic dosages to reach their optimal effects. Busrpirone is a long term anxiolytic that can be helpful in many of the anxiety disorders as well as anxiety associated with autism and Asperger's Syndrome. Although it is 'long acting' in the sense that it takes several weeks to reach therapeutic effects, it must be taken several times a day.

George had been in a terrible car accident. Ever since then, getting in any motor vehicle produced flashbacks of the accident and tremendous anxiety. He was placed on alprazolam (Xanax), twice a day for transportation to and from the day program. Xanax is approved by the FDA for use in panic disorders. It helped tremendously. Over time, however, staff noted that George was able to tolerate car rides to enjoyable places, even if he hadn't had the Xanax. (He only received it once on weekends). This gradual desensitization process combined with the medications allowed George to overcome his anxiety. Eventually staff felt that while he no longer appeared anxious in the car particularly, he seemed to have general problems all the time. The Xanax was switched over to clonazepam (Klonopin) which is a long acting benzodiazepam.

Within days, George was violently attacking others, and appeared very unhappy. The clonazepam was very disinhibiting for George. He was weaned off the clonazepam while staff monitored him to determine what course of action to take next. I saw him after he was weaned off the clonazepam. He was smiling, happy, and delighted to feel better. Staff had nothing but glowing reports to say about him. It seemed that for him, after treatment of his reactions to car rides, no medication was the best answer.

Alas, for many, many people, psychiatric illnesses are chronic. The medications help reduce the symptoms, but not cure the illness. PTSD is one of the very few that, with appropriate treatment, can be ameliorated. ('Cured' is not a term often seen in psychiatry at this time.)

5

Schizophrenia: The Split

Charles was one of the most distinguished persons that I have ever met. He was only 22 when we met, yet he had that kind of quiet confidence that you sense when you're with someone who knows his own worth. He didn't talk much, and that's what really bothered people. He was referred to me because people thought he was psychotic.

Charles has Down Syndrome. He lived in a group home that had been classified 'behavioral'. I met Charles in 1984 before the nature of psychiatric illnesses in persons with developmental disabilities was well understood. Even so, I never quite understood why he was in that particular home. His very silence made him stand out in a home where most of the people yelled. All of the other people in his home were aggressive or self destructive. Although Charles wasn't aggressive, he would occasionally put on a 50 cent plastic sheriff's badge and scribble in a notebook. After writing, he would "Humph" and put his things neatly away. Surely this was delusional, weird behavior.

Schizophrenia is the granddaddy of the psychiatric disorders. Historically, more people have been labelled schizophrenic than any other diagnosis. The accuracy of these diagnoses remains uncertain. People with disabilities have certainly been double labelled for years. Although the anti-psychotic medications continue to be the most commonly prescribed drugs for persons with developmental disabilities, schizophrenia is probably the least found disorder in this group.

What is schizophrenia? Unlike the bumper sticker

87

you may have read, "You're never alone when you're schizophrenic," the illness implies a split from reality, not a split personality or multiple personality disorder. Schizophrenia most often hits people in their late teens or early twenties. The disease can be very devastating to those individuals and their families. Most common is where a young person has been 'okay' in childhood. Some have always preferred to be alone, but overall they did well in school. Gradually, as the illness takes over, they become more isolative. They may become frightened of even familiar people. They no longer perform self-care, almost as if they no longer recognize the need for self-care. They may hear voices, and begin to firmly believe very bizarre things.

All of us have experienced illusions. An illusion is a misperception of a real stimulus. For example, on a hot day, the pavement may look wet. Or, if you've ever been alone in a house on a rainy night, you might think the wind in the trees was a burglar trying to break in. This is not psychotic. In each of these examples, other people could receive the same information through their own senses, and understand your misinterpretations.

Persons suffering from schizophrenia, however, are unable to trust their five senses. They may hear, see, taste, smell, or feel things that are not based in the real world. These are hallucinations. Hearing voices that no one else hears is the most common, but the hallucinations can involve any of the senses. Occasionally, the voices are friendly, but most often, the voices are very frightening to the person hearing them. Although the 'psychotic mass murderer' makes good newspaper headlines, it has been my experience that more people with schizophrenia are more afraid of the world than I need to be of them.

Persons suffering from this illness often experience

bizarre beliefs called delusions. A delusion, by definition, is a false fixed belief that no amount of logic can change. These beliefs may include that the television or radio has special messages just for them, that the secret police are following them, or that they have special magical powers. Often the delusions are of a paranoid nature: they believe that others are out to get them.

Imagine that you firmly believe that your next door neighbor is actually a foreign spy who is trying to kill you. You are highly unlikely to invite him over for coffee. No, you will try to avoid him at all costs. Now suppose that the people you live with try to convince you that the neighbor is simply a nice man. You would certainly begin to distrust the people you live with also. Thus the circle of mistrust grows, until it includes almost everyone you meet.

Whenever I work with someone who is psychotic (that is, experiencing delusions, and/or hallucinations), I always try to find out the nature of their delusions. Primarily, I am concerned to find out if they are a danger to themselves or others. Once that is done, I neither agree with their delusions, nor do I argue with them. By definition, a delusion is not swayed by other's logic. By agreeing with them, I deny their attempts to grasp reality. By arguing with them, I further their distrust in me. Typically, if a person appears frightened, I acknowledge their fear and try to help them feel safe. Remember, emotions are valid no matter their source.

With all people who experience delusions, the helper needs to work very hard to steer them to more reality based conversation, such as, what they had for breakfast or what is going on around you. Even when a person is very psychotic, not all of their person is out of reach. The person may still be able to discuss many subjects without problems. They may still have skills in music, art or sports. Build on these strengths.

In general, however, the sicker a person becomes the stranger their conversations. The person loses the ability to use abstract thinking. The standard test is to ask a person to explain a proverb such as 'people in glass houses shouldn't throw stones'. The person thinking concretely will answer, "You shouldn't throw stones because windows will break." When a person is admitted to a psychiatric hospital, I always asked, "What brought you here?" If the person began to explain about the problems they were having, I knew that person could think at least somewhat abstractly. A person with schizophrenia, however, would answer 'the bus', or 'the car'. This may be a difficult test for individuals with disabilities who, given the nature of the disability, have difficulty with abstraction. Here, I would have to know their ability to abstract and then test against their ability, rather than frustrate them by testing their disability.

Other changes in conversation will include tangential speech. The person with schizophrenia may string many sentences or even words together that are totally unrelated. The less amount of time that a person can talk on one subject, such as what they had for breakfast, the sicker they are. (Again, when reading this, remember that people with disabilities may have similar problems with speech that are related to the disability not to a disorder. It is important to know what they 'can' do and then measure it against what they 'are' doing.) The person may even make up their own words that have meaning only to them. The person may refuse to speak at all.

The facial expressions, or lack of them, of a person with schizophrenia can be very frightening to the lay

Characteristic Symptoms of Schizophrenia (DSM IV)

A) Two or more of the following:
   1) Delusions
   2) Hallucinations
   3) Disorganized speech
   4) Very disorganized behavior or total lack of movement (Catatonia)
   5) Negative symptoms (flat affect, inappropriate afect, lack of pleasure, poor eye contact, inability to initiate or persist in activities)
B) Social or occupational dysfuntion or very diminished self-care

person. We are used to getting feedback from the person we are speaking to via facial and body expressions. The person with schizophrenia has very little concept of abstract feeling states. Although the person may laugh or cry, often inappropriately (laugh when told their favorite relative died), their face shows little or no emotion. This is called flattening of affect. Any one of these symptoms alone is not enough to warrant a diagnosis of schizophrenia. It requires many of the attributes as outlined in Chart 5.1, and these 'symptoms' cannot be explained by other causes.

There are several different types of schizophrenia where one or more of the above symptoms are seen more prominently. The course, severity, and duration of any of these subtypes, can vary with the individual. Some people have a one time episode of schizophrenia that either spontaneously goes away (rarely), or is successfully treated with medications. Some people have periodic episodes of illness throughout their lives that require treatment. In between episodes, however, they are able to work and function. They may have residual difficulties, but over all, they are able to do okay. Unfortunately, some persons with schizophrenia, even with current treatment options, are never able to return to their pre-illness level of functioning.

There are many theories surrounding the cause of schizophrenia. The neurobiological theories look at neurotransmitters. The neurotransmitter said to be involved with schizophrenia is dopamine. It is believed that the nerve cells involved either excrete too much dopamine, or the receiving nerve cells are oversensitive to even normal amounts of dopamine. Studies are also beginning to show evidence that certain portions of the brain in persons with schizophrenia are structurally different. There are definite genetic correlates, in that persons with immediate family members with schizophrenia, have a higher than average chance of also developing the disease. Fortunately, 'bad' parenting is no longer seen as the cause of schizophrenia. (This will offer little comfort to parents who lived for years with the blame.)

Although there is research being conducted into the causes and treatments of schizophrenia, much more needs to be done. I suspect that part of the reason for the lack of definitive answers lies with the perceptions of schizophrenia itself. When my father had a heart attack from too much stress, it was acceptable for me to notify friends and family. People are much less likely to notify others and say, "Yeah, stress got to dad again, he's in the psych hospital." Psychiatric illnesses continue to be seen as evil, and somehow, the person's fault. Although schizophrenia effects far more people than AIDS, we don't see major fund raisers for psychiatric research.

Jack frustrated the people he lived and work with. Jack used to be able to navigate the bus system so well, he taught others in his home. Now, he won't leave his room. Jack was almost ready for his own apartment, but now he tells staff that 'a man in a white car' keeps following him. Jack used to have a job at a fast food restaurant that allowed him to buy a very fashionable wardrobe. The day we met he had on ripped shorts, two sweaters, and mismatched boots. He refused to change saying, "President Nixon wants me to wear these." Staff complained that Jack continually 'told stories.' Even as staff caught him in his 'lies,' he continued to tell his stories as if they were true. Jack had been on antipsychotics for years. Due to a pharmacy confusion, Jack had been receiving half his minimal dose for almost a month. His illness had returned.

Although Jack does have schizophrenia, many attributes of persons with disabilities have been misconstrued as symptoms of schizophrenia. For example, by definition, the developmental age of persons with developmental disabilities rarely exceeds 10-12 years of age. Abstract thinking does not develop in children until 12-14 years of age. This does NOT mean that disabled persons are unable to think, problem solve, or have insight. It simply means that their thinking will be on a different level. They will almost always give a concrete response to the proverb question. When a person develops schizophrenia, however, they lose the ability to think and communicate abstractly, and coherently. To diagnose a person with limited communication skills requires that someone else needs to be able to explain that there is a loss of function.

People may report to the psychiatrist that the person with developmental disabilities talks to himself. No one else can see who that person is talking to, well, this may or may not be a problem and it may or may not be psychotic. If you have children, have you ever heard yourself coming out of their mouths? We live out in the country. One night, I was making supper when my then 2 year old insisted, "Go outside, go outside!" I told her, "No she couldn't go because I'm making supper." Somehow I didn't want a 2 year old wandering out into the back field by herself. A little while later, I heard her talking. She had one of her dolls in her hands and said, "Go outside, go outside...No!" (I must have sounded a lot meaner than I intended.) What she was doing was replaying the situation over and over again. My refusing to let her go out was a situation that she found stressful. In role playing with her doll, she was able to work some things out for herself. People with disabilities may be doing the same thing.

My older child had a friend that came over and played all the time. This kid came over and played whenever my daughter wanted her to. The kid played whatever my daughter wanted to play. The child lost whatever game it was they were playing. In short, she was a perfect playmate. Eventually, my daughter exchanged her imaginary perfect friend for a real friend but she and her friends still act out life like situations just like she did with her invisible friend. Even now when she is bored or needs something to do, she creates somebody.

As I indicated before, we say people are developmentally delayed. They may still use coping strategies found at earlier levels of development. Now, we have individuals who talk to themselves, or at least it looks like they are talking to themselves because you don't see anyone else there. I suspect that if you really listen, you may hear them repeating things said to them or they may be replaying their day over to themselves.

Especially for the person living in a group situation who is bored or feels left out, you might hear him talk to a friend that no one else sees. This is not psychotic behavior. These behaviors may, in fact, be very useful for the individual. As the person grows, develops, and gains friends, and learns new ways to cope, these behaviors may disappear. Maybe not, I still talk to myself when I am busy working on a project. And some of the words I use have personal meanings and some may even be 'socially inappropriate.'

Another common complicating factor is when the person with developmental disabilities is experiencing flashbacks. The flashbacks of previously traumatic experiences may very well include 'visual or auditory hallucinations'. The person often fears that they are going crazy. Unfortunately, these sights and sounds are very reality based, old reality, but reality nevertheless. The use of anti-psychotic medications here may delay the healing process.

People wondered if Shelly was psychotic. She could often be found looking very frightened. During these times, she had a blank look on her face and would scream, "No, No!" Shelly was experiencing visual and auditory hallucinations of her past. Since several other concerns indicated the possibility of abuse, her past was reviewed. Not only had she been victimized in the institution, she had also been sexually abused by several family members prior to entering the institution. (She was originally placed in the institution when after years of abusing her, her family could no longer handle her 'sudden aggressive behavior!') Her hallucinations can better be understood as 'very real, very present, memories.'

Jack, unlike Shelly, clearly has schizophrenia. People could identify losses in function, however, indicators are seldom this clear. In general a diagnosis of schizophrenia should be considered as a last choice, not first, for safety's sake. Am I, therefore, declaring that there should be a total ban on anti-psychotic medications? No, not by a long shot. These medications are extremely important to those persons with schizophrenia and a few other psychotic disorders. These medications can have far reaching effects which are good when one considers how schizophrenia can debilitate many aspects of a person's life. I simply object to using a cannon when a fly swatter may be more effective.

It is said that the breakthrough in treatment for schizophrenia happened more by accident than design. There are several different stories, but all agree that the researchers were looking for medicines for other purposes when chlorpromazine was discovered. The scientists soon realized that chlorpromazine (Thorazine) helped to 'tranquilize' the insane.

If a little bit of something is good, then lots must be better. The average dose of Thorazine today is between 300 and 800 mg. per day for someone with active schizophrenia. In those days, people often received 1000 to 3000 mg, of this stuff. Remember in the 1950's, we still thought that the cause of schizophrenia was bad parenting and poor communication between parents and children. We thought that people with schizophrenia were experiencing very, very severe anxiety. Because these people slowed down, (I mean 1000 to 3000 mg of Thorazine would slow down a charging bull, for heaven's sake!) and seemed calmer somehow, we called these medications 'Major Tranquilizers'. In contrast, diazepam (Valium) was classified as a 'minor tranquilizer'. We had absolutely no comprehension of how these medications worked, in part because of our concept of the origin of schizophrenia.

Well, these medications somehow made their way over into the DD facilities. Persons with developmental disabilities suffered from various mental illnesses. They had suffered and were continuing to suffer from abusive situations. They were institutionalized and expected to be submissive, compliant, and quiet. The people rebelled with all sorts of normal responses to abnormal situations. They were placed on anti-psychotics in varying dosages for everything from trouble sleeping, to aggression.

Before I directly condemn the entire system, these medications did allow many people to be released from institutions. Unfortunately, the long term effects of the medicines were not at all understood. Eventually, we recognized that we could not continue to just 'chemically straitjacket' people. By the 1980's, we began to understand that schizophrenia had a biochemical nature. Since rapid reduction of these medications often brought on severe negative behaviors, we had to come up with diagnoses. We began to assess that they talk to themselves. They were aggressive. They yelled uncontrollably. They were aggressive. They use concrete thinking. They were aggressive. Sometimes their self-care was terrible. They were aggressive. They didn't sleep. They were aggressive. With all these things going on, well, they must be schizophrenic. And so, Schizophrenia or Psychotic Disorder, NOS (Not Otherwise Specified) became the number one psychiatric diagnosis for people with mental retardation.

At this time, if I work with someone with less than a high moderate range of mental retardation who is hearing voices, I'm very, very hesitant to ever label them with schizophrenia. The person has got to be able to conceptualize to me that the voices they are hearing are something that are not of this world. A typical conversation I have had with someone who is thought to be schizophrenic, sounds like this:

"Do you hear voices?"

"Yes!"

"Whose voice are you hearing?"

"Your's."

"No, no, no. Are you hearing any voices of somebody who is not here in this room?"

"Yes."

"Whose voices are you hearing?"

"The people in the room next door."

When I finally get down to, "Is this voice that you are hearing something that anybody else could hear if they were sitting here?" The results become questionable because the questions have necessarily become abstract in order to get away from concrete thinking related to the developmental disability. It then becomes paramount to look for some of the other symptomatology that goes with schizophrenia such as the regression of self-care, the difficulty dealing with other people, the flattened affect, and delusional thinking. And just to complicate issues, remember, that just because you may not understand what a person is saying, does not make the ideas delusional. More simply put, the person may be relaying factual information that others do not want to hear. (Talking about abusive episodes, behavior of staff or other subjects uncomfortable for the listener, but a reality for the speaker.)

Many people will ask, "If the person is aggressive, and the anti-psychotic seems to control it somewhat, why is using these medications such a big deal?" How many of you would shoot me if I wanted to take someone off an anti-psychotic medication? Let's be honest. How many of you think that the person in question, based on the above criteria, is really and truly schizophrenic? What is the fear or the real concern of what could happen when they come off the medication? "The person will be aggressive!"

The anti-psychotic medications (now called 'neuroleptic' rather than 'major tranquilizers') as a group are dopamine blockers. If you can recall back to the highly technical drawing of the neurons, (Chart 3.3) the neurotransmitters bind in the next cells' receptors (receivers). The anti-psychotics fill in the dopamine receptor spots, so that Dopamine cannot activate the next cell. In this way, for the person with schizophrenia, even though the cells either produce too much dopamine, or are hypersensitive to dopamine, the next cell is not triggering when it should.

(For a list of neuroleptic medications, see Chart 5.2a and 5.2b)

When this blockade is put into effect in a person without schizophrenia, the brain cells are really compromised especially for a person with cognitive difficulties. Normal signals for thinking, feeling, reasoning, and understanding the world around them are reduced. It's sort of like someone telling you to sort dark socks by color and then turning out the lights!

Besides decreased cognition, the anti-psychotics as a group are not very specific and can create many side effects even in those persons who do need these medications. Unfortunately, the dopamine blockers cannot (at this time) distinguish between which type of dopamine receptors they should block and which ones they shouldn't. In addition to this, they are not 'pure' medications such that they also block other receptor sites besides the dopamine ones. Consequently, they create many side effects, neurological and otherwise.

If the person is not schizophrenic and receives anti-psychotic medications, they may suffer unnecessarily from devastating side effects that can effect anyone (including those people with schizophrenia). Tardive dyskinesia (TD) is an often irreversible side effect of most of the anti-psychotic medications. TD usually develops after the person had been taking the medication for extended periods of time. Some people even develop TD after only a very short time on the medication. Ironically, however, the very medications that create this movement disorder also mask it to some extent.

TD generally begins with movements of the tongue,

mouth, and jaw. Particularly when the person is relaxing, you will notice that they look like they are chewing a very large piece of gum. They may scrunch up their lips, or smack their lips together. The person may also make a pill-rolling motion of the fingers. Some people develop movements throughout their entire body.

My best friend is also a nurse. She's a 'real nurse' and works in a hospital. She called me one day about a woman who is on the orthopaedic floor (bones). This elderly woman fell and broke her hip and they needed to put her in traction. Now you need to understand, part of the reason that I work in psychiatry is because I avoid all that other stuff. So I asked, "Why are you calling me?" She replied that someone had abruptly discontinued her anti-psychotic medication that she had been on for years. They were wondering if that might have had something to do with her fall.

After the medication was stopped, this woman began having entire body gyrations that were out of her control as a result of tardive dyskinesia. These gyrations caused her to fall and break her hip in the first place, and were preventing her from benefitting from traction in the second place. She had to be placed back on even higher doses of the anti-psychotic until the hip healed.

Other common side effects associated with the high potency anti-psychotics (those anti-psychotics that only require 1-40 milligrams to achieve the desired responses) are the extrapyramidal side effects (EPS). No, the person does not develop an urge to go to Egypt and erect triangular structures. These are motor movement side effects. Dopamine receptors are also located in the nervous pathways associated with movement. When the blockade effects this system, you may see one or more of the following: akathisia,

Parkinson's, and dystonic movements.

Have you ever been sitting at a table with one or more people who have had too much caffeine? Their legs get shaking so hard that they can literally cause the table to shake. I remember having had so much caffeine prior to an exam, that I had the whole row of desks moving. Other testers were not happy with me. This is mild compared to the akathisia associated with dopamine blockers. The person may dance from foot to foot. They may pace restlessly. The person may report feeling very anxious. Some times we misdiagnose the restlessness as a need for more medications, and increase their dosage which compounds the problem.

Interestingly, some people develop Parkinsonian syndrome where they appear to have Parkinson's disease. (Parkinson's disease is caused from too little dopamine in the movement pathways) The person develops mask-like faces (hard to observe in someone with a flat affect!), resting tremors, rigid posture, and a shuffling walk.

Dystonia involves the muscles of the eye, neck and/or throat. The person's eyes may move up in the socket and not come down. The neck area may swell, become stiff, and even close off the airway for breathing! The EPS side effects can be relieved by also prescribing 'antiparkinsonism' medications such as benztropine (Cogentin), amantadine (Symmetrel), diphenhydramine (Benedryl), or trihexyphenidyl (Artane). Unfortunately, these medications also have their own side effects most notably, the anticholinergic side effects that are also seen in the low potency anti-psychotics. (Those anti-psychotics that require 100-1000 mgs. to achieve the desired response).

The anticholinergic side effects are most commonly

Chart 5.2a

Antipsychotic/Neuroleptic Medications

LOW POTENCY

	DOSAGE RANGE[1]	EPS [2,3]	ANTI-C [2,4]
chlorpromazine (Thorazine)	300 - 800 mg/day	X	XXX
chlorprothixene (Taractin)	200 - 600 mg/day	X	XXX
thioridazine (Mellaril)	100 - 600 mg/day	X	XXX

INTERMEDIATE POTENCY

acetophenazine (Tindal)	20 - 100 mg/day	XX	XX
loxapine (Loxitane)	10 - 250 mg/day	XX	XX
molidone (Moban)	50 - 225 mg/day	XX	XX
perphenazine (Trilafon)	4 - 64 mg/day	XX	XX
mesoridazine (Serentil)	25 - 200 mg/day	XX	XX

HIGH POTENCY

fluphenazine (Prolixin)	1 - 20 mg/day	XXX	X
haloperidol (Haldol)	1 - 20 mg/day	XXX	X
pimozide (Orap)	1 - 10 mg/day	XXX	X
thiothixene (Navane)	1 - 20 mg/day	XXX	X
trifluoperazine (Stelazine)	2 - 20 mg/day	XXX	X

---

[1] Actual dosage range for an individual will vary to age, diagnosis, and symptoms.
[2] X= Occasionally   XX= Often   XXX= Very Often
[3] Extrapyramidal Side Effects: akathesia, Parkinsonism, and/ or dystonia.
[4] Anticholinergic Side Effects:
Drowsiness, constipation, blurry vision, delayed urination, sexual dysfunctions, and/or dry mouth.

Chart 5.2b

Antipsychotic/Neuroleptic Medications [Continued]
New Antipsychotics

	Average Dosage Range	Cautions
clozapine (Clozaril)	50 - 600 mg/day	Potential for lowered white blood cell count requires weekly blood draws. May cause sedation, dizziness, low blood pressure, drooling, and/or constipation. Not associated with T.D.
risperidone (Risperdal)	0.5 - 16 mg/day	Side effects increase as dosage increases

List of Antipsychotics available in Canada, but not the United States:[5]

> fluphenthixol (Fluanxol)
> fluspiriline (Imap)
> methotrimeprazine (Nozinan, Leuoprome)
> thioproperazine (Mejeptil)

Other Side Effects:

Tardive Dyskinesia associated with all antipsychotics except perhaps clozapine. Increased susceptability to sunburn, rash, blood disorders, hormone changes (some women stop having periods but can still get pregnant!), and breast enlargement in both men and women. Thioridazine is associated with increased pigment in the eyes which can lead to blindness. Neuroleptic Malignant Syndrome is a rare but dangerous effect of these medications - - symptoms include extreme rigidity, high fever, rapid heart rate and breathing, heavy sweating, and/or confusion. Requires immediate emergency intervention.

---

[5] The author has never worked with these medications and is not qualified to provide other information.

seen with the low potency anti-psychotics such as Thorazine and Mellaril. These side effects include constipation, blurred vision, dry mouth, drowsiness, low energy, sensitivity to the sun, lowered sexual drive and abilities to reach orgasm, and many others. Some of these side effects ease up over time, or perhaps the person learns to live with these feelings over time. My experience has been that these side effects are more keenly noted by those persons without actual schizophrenia.

I realize that I have just used many medical terms with few revealing illustrations. In part, because it is important to realize that while these medications are invaluable to the person with schizophrenia, they are not taken without significant price tags (negative side effects on the body). This is the best way I know to answer the question of, "So what's wrong with giving these medicines if it controls aggression?"

Staff brought Amanda in for a psychiatric consult. She was diagnosed with profound mental retardation, a Hepatitis B carrier, and many, many negative behaviors. She spit, she screamed, she attacked others, and scratched herself to the point where she bled. I met her before I had a real understanding of the next concept. The hate mail that I received from staff was justifiable.

Amanda's community doctor had been maintaining the 250 mg. per day of thioridazine (Mellaril) that she had received for years in the institutions. He requested a psychiatric consult to see if the medication was still necessary. As I could recognize no symptoms of psychosis in this woman, the thioridazine seemed unnecessary. Unfortunately, although she was not psychotic, the Mellaril covered up some of the more noticeable symptoms of the major depression that she did have. The community doctor abruptly discontinued the Mellaril. A month later, Amanda came unglued. Staff hated me.

Have you ever taken a 'non' non drowsy cold tablet (the kind that makes you sleepy) by mistake and then tried to work? That feeling of being in a cloud is what persons taking anti-psychotic medications often feel like. We then expect these people to go to their workshops and sort widgets by the hour. Amanda had been under this cloud for years. When the medication was abruptly stopped, she experienced neuroleptic withdrawal syndrome.

Neuroleptic Withdrawal Syndrome is highlighted by the person having a massive rebound effect to their own neurotransmitters when the medications are stopped. The idea is that neurons which are experiencing dopamine blockade from the anti-psychotic medications adapt by becoming oversensitive to whatever dopamine they receive. When the dopamine blockade is removed abruptly (more than 20% of the anti-psychotic discontinued at a time), the receptors are freed up and react violently to all the 'excess' dopamine. We literally create temporary illness in these people.

Usually, you will not notice this effect right away. The anti-psychotic medications cause a person to put on excess body fat, and then the medicine stores itself in body fat. This fat-stored medicine is slowly used up, so that you will generally not notice symptoms of withdrawal until 3-4 weeks later. (This also explains why a person with actual schizophrenia will feel like they do not need the medicines, because they can often go for days without serious problems. Unfortunately, by the time the medicines have slowly left their body, they have often had a major decompensation.)

106

Common recommendations now are that no more than 10-20% of the medication should be decreased every 2 - 6 months. The actual taper process varies from person to person, and how long they have been receiving the medications.

Often times while the medications are being decreased, symptoms of the probable original psychiatric or other medical illness are revealed (as in Amanda's case, the depression became evident). Since many people who are non-verbal act out their symptoms, you may well see an increase in aggression. THIS DOES NOT MEAN THAT YOU SHOULD ALWAYS RESTART THE ANTI-PSYCHOTIC!!! It means, you should also look at the other symptoms to see what other diagnosis may be more appropriate and treat accordingly. You may see the rare person experience a true psychotic decompensation with this process, but it has definitely been more the exception than the rule.

Elizabeth had been receiving over 500 mg. of Thorazine a day for over 15 years. She always had problems with constipation . One day she became so constipated that she developed an obstructed bowel. The doctor in the hospital immediately discontinued the Thorazine. She was in the hospital for complications of the obstructed bowel for weeks. By the time she returned home, most of the severe withdrawal symptoms had subsided. Although it had undoubtedly been a horrendous time for her, no one wanted to restart the Thorazine. Although no psychiatric symptoms emerged, staff noted that she cried more around her periods. Medical follow-up revealed that she had been suffering from very painful gynaecological problems for years. She is now receiving more appropriate treatment for what was probably the difficulty all along.

Remember Charles with the sheriff's badge? Since I was supposed to assess Charles, we set up a plan of going out to area restaurants once a week. He always held my car door, and the restaurant door. He did let me order for myself, but he always insisted on carrying the tray. Some might call Charles chauvinistic, but I loved every minute of it. He was a shy guy, but over time, we developed an enjoyable camaraderie.

One day, he told me about the night his mom's house was broken into. I had long since realized that Charles had an absolute sense of right and wrong. There were no grays for him. It really bothered him when anyone violated the rules. Anyway, as he told me about the break in, he relayed the incident like it had just happened when in fact it had occurred years ago. He said that the police came to the house and took a report. His mom told him, "Everything will be alright. The police took a report, and that took care of everything." "Humpf." As he said that, a light went off in my head. Whenever someone violated the rules of the group home, which in his house happened a lot, he put on his badge and wrote a report to right the wrong. Charles had a greater grasp of reality than many people I know, he never was psychotic.

6
So Now What?

I was in a rush to get to work. I grabbed a brand new outfit for my three year old. She screamed, "NNNOOO!!! It doesn't spin!" She likes her dresses to have full skirts so when she turns around they 'spin'. I was very close to holding her down and forcing it on her. Common sense prevailed. (Common sense meant that my older daughter found another dress and she convinced the younger one that it 'spinned'. I was still in a mood to force the new outfit over her head!)

Some things in life are not a choice. I might want to drive on the wrong side of the road, but I can't. In no way should such behavior be condoned. There are many things over which we do not have control, nor do we give choices. For example, I do not ask my children if they want their immunizations. No child wants a shot, but that is not a time when I offer a choice. After the shot is completed, however, I might let them choose a favorite treat for having gone through it.

Responsible adults learn by having a lifetime of making both good and bad decisions. You can learn from both situations. Most educators will agree that allowing children to make their own decisions increases learning and self-esteem. We haven't often allowed people with developmental disabilities to have a choice. This is dangerous for many reasons. There is no possible way we can teach a person to say the big "NO's" to unwanted touch or unwanted medications, when we won't even allow them to say the little "No's", to unwanted broccoli for supper. If we don't allow people to make choices, legitimate choices, and respect that choice, we are no better than any other slave owner (or me on a hurried morning!). By definition a choice means that there is a true freedom to decide.

We may find that a lot of the 'negative behaviors' go away, just because we start treating the choices that people with disabilities make with respect. Respect means that we don't try to rewrite the treatment plan when their choice isn't what we deem to be in their best interest. We may never need medication, if we simply get rid of some of the blocks that have been put in peoples' lives. Staff knew Harvey was depressed. They reported that he looked sad and was refusing food he had always eaten. On closer examination, staff at his day program had been respecting more and more of his choices. The contrast of the overwhelming lack of choices in his home was making Harvey sad and frustrated. He had lost no weight, but he was refusing to eat fish, Brussels sprouts and rice. Since I'm not a fan of fish or Brussels sprouts myself, I took this as a true sign of the intelligence I always suspected he had rather than a psychiatric emergency. A change in homes and continued encouragement and respect for choices were far more prescriptive than any anti-depressant for Harvey.

These past few chapters have only begun to skim the surface of information becoming available on dual diagnosis. Although this covers the basics, it doesn't fine tune information for persons with various disorders such as Autism, Asperger's Syndrome, Fetal Alcohol Syndrome, Fragile X or any of the other new 'flavors' of disability being discovered. There are no medication 'cures' for these disorders, but sometimes common symptoms can be helped with medication.

Kevin has autism. He insists on absolute sameness for everything. The same route must be taken to day program. The same cereal must be eaten for breakfast. Only he can sit in the blue chair. If it's 7:00p.m., he must be watching 'Star Trek' reruns. If anyone violates these 'rules', he becomes very aggressive. Although this insistence on sameness is common in persons with autism, it severely debilitated him in a world not known for sameness. Fluoxetene (Prozac) has helped him deal with changes. He continues to have trouble relating to people, he still has problems communicating, he still twirls objects. He no longer hits himself, however, when the van stops at the store on the way home from work.

People are not just the sum total of their parts, but a connected being that is finely tuned by both positive and negative events, conditions, and people in their lives. I hope that the reader has come to understand that to say a person is aggressive, is only to start the process. Aggression can be seen as a form of communication. Perhaps the person has a psychiatric disorder. Perhaps she is frightened. Perhaps he has a stomach ulcer. Perhaps, perhaps, perhaps....

People sometimes argue that even if a person could be helped by appropriate medications given for real mental illnesses, why handicap the person further by giving them extra negative labels. Do all these extra psychiatric labels hurt? Perhaps, sometimes. If you remember my shopping expeditions, you can probably figure out that designer labels on clothes mean very little to me. Although I appreciate fine quality and workmanship, paying extra only to carry someone else's name, doesn't make sense to me; neither do labels that are used simply to further alienate people. On the other hand, if I removed all the labels from the canned goods in my kitchen, meals at our home would be more of an adventure than they already are. Imagine taking two unlabelled cans and mixing them together -- such as cherry pie filling and vegetable soup? (My husband is convinced I cook this way anyway!)

If a person with an unlabelled psychiatric diagnosis is prescribed 'the drug of the month', heaven knows what will happen. In some cases the mix might work, but more often the results would be horrible. In situations such as this, labels, or correct diagnoses if you will, are essential, not luxuries or hindrances.

Labels, or diagnoses, are important for other medical treatments as well. Knowing that a person has Down Syndrome tells me that I should be monitoring for hypothyroidism. (Approximately 30% of persons with Down Syndrome will also develop hypothyroidism and need annual screening for this.) Often the first symptoms may include depression, lethargy, cold intolerance, dry skin, or confusion. Untreated hypothyroidism can lead to permanent decline of mental functions.

How would you feel if you were mislabelled? We used to live in Detroit and my husband started a new job several hours away. I was 4 months pregnant when he left. I had to finish teaching a nursing course at the college, had the care of our 4 year old, and had to sell our house. While all of this was going on, my father had another heart attack and had to have quadruple by-pass surgery. He was in intensive care for over three weeks. Needless to say, there was a little bit of stress going on in our lives.

We finally moved into our new house over the Memorial Day weekend. Now, I've read the DD handbook. Remember what I said, things only happen on a holiday weekend. The baby was pressing on the sciatic nerve in my left leg. It was very painful for me. In fact, my leg would give out from underneath me. After a couple of days of all the moving, I was in misery.

One of our dogs was in a kennel about an hour drive from our house. My husband ever so kindly (I think he was tired of listening to me complain) said, "Sue go get the dog. Take a nice slow drive, so you can relax and feel better." Nice thought! I go to get the dog. As I'm walking out of the people's house, the baby pushed on my sciatic nerve. My left leg went out from under me. I fell and broke my right foot in two places. I was an hour from our new house. Our new phone was not installed yet. Our health insurance didn't travel to the town I was currently in. I have the four year old with me. I've worked in this field long enough to know what happens when you fall on a baby at 6 months' gestation.

When I got to the hospital, my blood pressure was very high from the combined pain, fear, and long term stress. (Normally, my blood pressure ran around 80/50 while I was pregnant.)

If I were non-verbal, I could not have explained to somebody about the pain in my foot. I could not have explained about my concerns for my baby. I could not have reached my husband for support. If the only thing that the emergency room staff did was to check my blood pressure and saw that it was high, they might have labelled me as having high blood pressure and given me some type of medication to bring my blood pressure down and sent me home. Now, a few days after that, my foot would have still been very, very sore, but not as painful. Some of my current concerns about the baby may have subsided as I felt it kick. If my blood pressure went back to 80/50 and I was on a medication that lowered my blood pressure, I would have become very sick, possibly even died. It certainly would have harmed the baby. My foot would have never gotten fixed.

A few years back and even as recent as within the last three days, somebody has been placed on an anti-psychotic such as Mellaril or Haldol for a 'broken foot.' We need to recognize that perhaps she's depressed. We need to acknowledge that perhaps he has been violently sexually abused for years. Instead, we found the medications that covered things up and didn't recognize what the long term ramifications of that would be. Now we have opportunities for change.

"When the day of Pentecost came, all the believers were gathered together in one place. Suddenly there was a noise from the sky which sounded like a strong wind blowing, and it filled the whole house where they were sitting. Then they saw what looked like tongues of fire which spread out and touched each person there. They were all filled with the Holy Spirit and began to talk in other languages, as the spirit enabled them to speak."

Acts 2, 1-4

I firmly believe that only the Supreme Being can bring such different languages together, and S/He hasn't seen fit to blend all mental health agencies into one 'supremely' well functioning unit. (I suspect some miracles are far more difficult than others!) The "Psychiatric Tower of Babble" however, has not been about faith. The psychiatric medications are not manna provided from gods. Psychiatry is not a religion. Mental health professionals are not priests that can look in their crystal balls and solve all things. Maybe, just maybe, however, if one more person is helped because those who care about him can now speak the same language as the psychiatrist, maybe I've paid some of the debt back that I owe Joe. Maybe not.

You will recall Joe from the first chapter. He was the gentleman whose younger brother was also named Joe. I was 18 when we met. I knew even less about developmental disabilities than I did about cooking meals for 20 people. I discovered the group home when I was picking up some carpet samples for my parents. Both the owner of the group home and my parents were having houses built by the same guy. I needed a summer job, the group home needed a staff person.

Three years ago, Joe had been moved to his home from the institution with his lifelong friend, Kenny. Joe followed the same routine, every morning. First, he woke up when his cheap, blue, wind-up alarm clock went off at 6:30. Joe could not tell time. He relied on others to regulate the clock to the right time, but he never failed to set the alarm at night. If he forgot to set his alarm, he wouldn't have enough time to help Kenny. Kenny also had Down Syndrome, but he had more physical challenges than Joe did. Joe had been helping Kenny get up, dressed, and groomed for over 35 years. Kenny relied on Joe. Joe relied on his clock.

After getting himself and Kenny ready for the day, Joe would always come downstairs and say "I 'ike you." "I like you too, Joe." We would both smile and continue our mornings.

I was running errands for the home in my car one

day. Joe came along to keep me company. He pointed to all the dials on my car wanting to know what they were for. He noted that one spot was empty. I explained that it was a spot for a clock, but my car didn't have one. (In 1977, cars still needed a 4" diameter hole on the dash for a clock, not a 1" square for digital numbers on the radio.)

The next day, Joe came downstairs for his usual "I 'ike you." Instead of leaving after my response, however, he insisted that I follow him. Sitting on the dash of my car was a cheap, blue, wind-up alarm clock. Now, my car had a clock too.

I never wind it up because it ticks, but I am never without it. Thanks again, Joe. I like you too.

REFERENCES AND RESOURCES

Aman, M. & Arnold, L.E. (1991). Beta Blockers in Mental Retardation and Developmental Disorders. Journal of Child and Adolescent Psychopharmacology (1) 5, p. 361-373.

American Psychiatric Association, 1994. Diagnostic and Statistical Manual of Mental Disorders, 4th Ed. Washington D.C.: American Psychiatric Association

Arnold, L.E. (1993). Clinical Pharmacological Issues in Treating Psychiatric Disorders of Patients with Mental Retardation. Annals of Clinical Psychiatry, 51, p.189-198.

Cole, S.S. (1984-1986). Facing the Challenges of Sexual Abuse in Persons with Disabilities. Sexuality and Disability, 7(314), p. 71-88.

Coulter, D.L. (1993). Epilepsy and Mental Retardation, American Journal on Mental Retardation, Vol. 98, Supplement, p. 1-11.

Cushna, B., Szymanski, L.S., & Tanguey, P.E. (1980). Professional Roles and Unmet Manpower Needs. In L.S. Szymanski and P.E. Tanguay (Eds.) Emotional Disorders of Mentally Retarded Persons. Baltimore: University Park Press.

Drooker M.A., Byck R., (1992). Physical Disorders Presenting as Psychiatric Illness: A New View. The Psychiatric Times (7). p.19-24.

Eaton, L.F. & Menolascino, F.J. (1982). Psychiatric Disorders in the Mentally Retarded: Types, Problems and Challenges. American Journal of Psychiatry. (139) 10, p.1297-1303.

Fidura, J., Lindsey, R., & Walker, G. (1987). A Special Behavior Unit for Treatment of Behavior Problems of Persons Who are

Mentally Retarded. Mental Retardation (25) 2, p. 107-111.

Gedye, A. (1992). Recognizing Obsessive-Compulsive Disorder in Clients With Developmental Disabilities. The Habilitative Mental Healthcare Newsletter (11) 11, p. 73-77.

Good News Bible (1976). New York: American Bible Society.

Hingsburger, D. (1989). Relationship Training, Sexual Behavior, and Persons with Developmental Handicaps. The Habilitative Healthcare Newsletter, (8) 5.

Jacobson, J.W. & Janicki, M.P. (1987). Needs for Professional and Generic Services Within a Developmental Disabilities Care System. In J.A. Mulick & R.F. Antonak (Eds). Transitions in Mental Retardation (Vol. 2): Issues in Therapeutic Intervention (pp. 23-46) Norwood J.J.: Ablex.

Lakin, K., Hill, B., Hauber, F., Bruinintis, R. & Heal, L. (1983). New Admissions and Readmissions to a National Sample of Public Residential Facilities. American Journal of Mental Deficiency (88) p. 13-20.

Lansdell, C. (1990). Psychotherapy with Persons Who Have Developmental Disabilities: A Bio-psycho-social model. The NADD Newsletter (7) 2, p. 1,4-5.

Lasalandra, M. (1995). Group Home OK'D Despite Death. The Boston Herald, Wed. Feb. 15, 1995

Levitas, A., McCandless, G., Reid, C., Sobel, B., & Elenewski, E. (1993). Behavioral and Psychiatric Phenotypes in Five Mental Retardation Syndromes. In Celebrating a Decade of Excellence. Philidelphia: NADD 10th Annual Conference proceedings, p. 71-73

Ludwig, S., Hingsburger, D. (1989). Preparartion for Counseling and Psychotherapy: Teaching About Feelings. Psychiatric aspects of mental retardation reviews (8) 1. p.1-7

Myers, B.A., & Pueschel, S.M. (1993). Differentiating Schizophrenia From Other Mental and Behavioral Disorders in Persons with Developmental Disabilities. The Habilitative Mental Healthcare Newsletter (12) 6, p. 93-98.

Medical Economics Data Production Co. (1995). Physicians Desk Reference (PDR) 45th Edition Montvale, NJ: Author

Poindexter, A. (1993). Can Depakote or Tegretol Change My Life? Behavioral Consequences of Simplified Antiepileptic Drug Regimes. The NADD Newsletter (11) 3, P.1-3.

Reiss, S. (1982). Psychopathology and Mental Retardation: Survey of a Developmental Disabilities Mental Health Program. Mental Retardation, (20) 3, p. 128-132.

Reiss, S. (1988). Dual Diagnosis in the United States. Australia and New Zealand Journal of Developmental Disabilities, (14) 3, p. 43-48.

Reiss, S. & Benson, B.A. (1984). Awareness of Negative Social Conditions Among Mentally Retarded, Emotionally Disturbed Outpatients. American Journal of Psychiatry, (141), p. 88-90.

Reiss, S. & Benson, B.A. (1985). Psychosocial Correlates of Depression in Mentally Retarded Adults: I. Minimal Social Supports and Stigmatization. American Journal of Mental Deficiency, (89) 4, p. 331-337.

Ryan, R., Rodden P.J., & Sunada K.A., (1991). A Model for Interdisciplinary On Site Evaluation of People Who Have "Dual Diagnosis". The NADD Newsletter,(8)1, 1-4.

Ryan, R. (1993). Medication Management of Post Traumatic Stress Disorder in Persons With Developmental Disabilities. In Celebrating a Decade of Excellence Philipelphia: 10th Annual Conference N.A.D.D. p. 1-3

Ryan, R. (1994). Asperger's Syndrome. The Habilitative Mental

Healthcare Newsletter (13) 1, p. 1-6.

Sobsey, D. (1994). The Research that Shattered the Myths: Understanding the Incidence and Nature of Abuse and Abusers. The NADD Newsletter (11) 3, p. 1-4.

Sobsey D., Gray S., Pyper D., & Reimer-Heck B., (1991) Disability, Sexuality, and Abuse, An Annotated Bibliography. Baltimore: Paul H. Brookes Publishing Co.

Sovner, R. & Hurley, A. (1989). Ten Diagnostic Principles for Recognizing Psychiatric Disorders in Mentally Retarded Persons. Psychiatric Aspects of Mental Retardation Reviews (8) 2, p. 9-14.

Sovner, R. & Hurley, A. (1990). Affective Disorder Update. The Habilitative Mental Health Care Newsletter (9) 12, p. 103-108.

Tharinger, Horton, & Miller (1990). Sexual Abuse and Exploitation of Children and Adults with Mental Retardation and Other Handicaps. Child Abuse and Neglect (14), p. 301-312.

Weber, L., & Wimner, S. (1986). Mental Illness in persons with mental retardation: ARC Facts, Arlington, Texas: Association for Retarded Citizens.

Yudofsky, S.C., Hales, R.E., & Ferguson, T. (1991). What You Need to Know About Psychiatric Drugs. New York: Ballantine Publishers.

About the Author

Sue Gabriel is a Psychiatric Nurse Practitioner for a large midwestern community health center. She has her Master's Degree in Psychiatric Nursing from the University of Michigan and is a certified clinical specialist. She has written for several professional journals. Ms Gabriel provides clinical consultations and conducts conferences in dual diagnosis. Her career has focused on direct clinical work with persons with developmental disabilities and/or psychiatric illness as well as instructing undergraduate and graduate nursing students.

Persons wishing to contact Ms. Gabriel may do so through Diverse City Press or by contacting her at Community Support Services, 407 W. Greenlawn, Lansing MI, 48910; (517) 374-8000.

About Diverse City Press

Diverse City Press has set a goal of publishing vital, insightful, yet affordable material for persons in the field of developmental disability. We are open to comments regarding all of our published books and videos as well as open to receiving manuscripts from people who work directly in the field of developmental disabilities.

Other Products Available Through Diverse City Press

JUST SAY KNOW! BY DAVE HINGSBURGER. This book explores the victimization of people with disabilities and suggests new ways to understand and reduce the risk of sexual assault.

Nurturing Dreams and Celebrating Success: This two hour audiotape is a live recording of Dave Hingsburger speaking on the issue of self esteem in regards to people with developmental disabilities. Lively and funny!!

I OPENERS By Dave Hingsburger This book is a question/answer book written for parents about sexuality and developmental disability.

UNDER COVER DICK. TEACHING MEN WITH DISABILITIES ABOUT CONDOM USE THROUGH UNDERSTANDING AND VIDEO. This book and video by Dave Hingsburger provides a tool to teach about condom use as well as suggest how our service needs to change. Safe sex means more than just not getting caught.

HAND MADE LOVE A GUIDE FOR TEACHING ABOUT MALE MASTURBATION THROUGH UNDER-STANDING AND VIDEO. BY DAVE HINGSBURGER. This book and video set provides facts about masturbation in human service and an education tool for teaching and reducing anxiety.

Behaviour Self! This book by Dave Hingsburger looks at how behaviour communicates and suggests new tools for 'listening' and for responding.

Quantity	Title	Unit Price	TOTAL
	Just Say Know!	$16 CAN$ 14 US	
	Behaviour Self!	$16 CAN$ 14 US	
	Hand Made Love	Book only $16 CAN$ 14 US video set $50 CAN$ 40 US	
	Under Cover Dick	Book & video set $50 CAN$ 40 US	
	I-Openers	$16 CAN$ 14 US	
	Nurturing Dreams (Audio)	$25 CAN$23 US	
		TOTAL	$

NAME:_____

ORGANIZATION:_____

STREET ADDRESS:_____

CITY:_____ PROV(STATE)_____

POSTAL(ZIP) CODE:_____

Diverse City Press
BM 272, 33 des Floralies
Eastman, QC
Canada
J0E 1P0

The Habilitative Mental Healthcare Newsletter

A Bimonthly Mental Health / Mental Retardation Publication

In many agencies this is the most often read journal by staff at every level of involvement with people with developmental disabilities. This journal gives insightful and *useable* information.

Current subscription rates:

US $49 personal
$63 institutional

Canada/Mexico $58 personal
$74 institutional

Psych-media, Inc.
PO Box 57
Bear Creek, NC
27207-0057   tel (910) 581-3700
                    fax (910) 581-3766